Distance Education in Nursing

Karen H. Frith, PhD, RN, NEA-BC, is a professor of nursing at the University of Alabama in Huntsville. From 2002 to 2007 she was the chair of graduate nursing at Georgia College & State University. She has been a nurse educator for 20 years and began teaching online in 1995. She is a member of the American Organization of Nurse Executives (AONE), served on the distance education national committee of the American Association of Colleges of Nursing, and is a member in many other nurse organizations. She serves as a reviewer (grants and articles) for Sigma Theta Tau, Health Resources and Services Administration, *Journal of Issues in Nursing Education*, *Journal of Health & Medical Informatics*, *Journal of Nursing Education*, and *Journal of Nursing Administration*, among others. She has authored 27 articles in peer-reviewed journals and 3 book chapters and presents nationally. Previous clinical positions include nurse manager of cardiovascular surgical intensive care at the Medical Center of Central Georgia, with a decade of experience as a staff nurse. She is board certified by the American Nurses Credentialing Center as Nurse Executive, Advanced (NEA-BC).

Deborah J. Clark, PhD, MSN, MBA, RN, CNE, is the online BSN program director at ECPI University in Virginia Beach, Virginia. She has been an associate dean for nursing, director of nurses, and associate professor of nursing at Georgia College & State University. She is a nurse educator with 17 years of teaching experience both in seat and online. She is a member of the National League for Nursing (NLN) and a National League for Nursing Accrediting Commission (NLNAC) program evaluator, and serves as a reviewer for the *Online Journal of Issues in Nursing* and *Computers, Informatics & Nursing*. She has authored 10 journal articles and developed the Internet Consequences Scales (ICONS) with Dr. Frith. Dr. Clark is a Certified Nurse Educator. Prior to beginning her teaching career, Dr. Clark held clinical positions in surgical ICU and neurological, renal, and long-term care.

Distance Education in Nursing

Third Edition

Karen H. Frith, PhD, RN, NEA-BC

Deborah J. Clark, PhD, MSN, MBA, RN, CNE

Editors

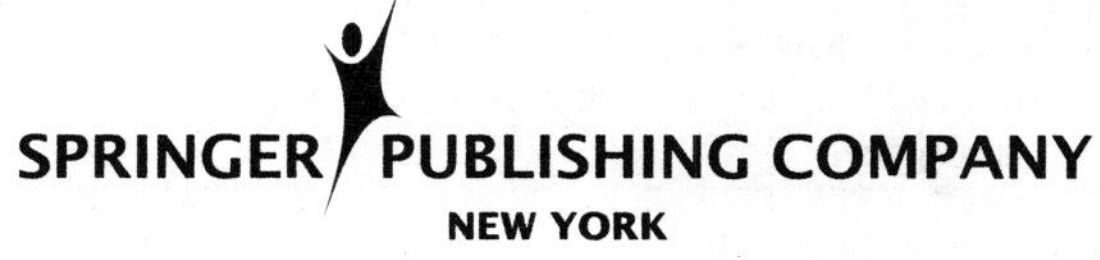

Springer Publishing Company, LLC
11 West 42nd Street
New York, NY 10036
www.springerpub.com

Acquisitions Editor: Allan Graubard
Production Editor: Joseph Stubenrauch
Composition: Manila Typesetting Company

ISBN: 978-0-8261-0945-3
E-book ISBN: 978-0-8261-0046-0

12 13 14 15/ 5 4 3 2 1

Library of Congress Cataloging-in-Publication Data
Distance education in nursing.—3rd ed. / Karen H. Frith, Deborah J. Clark, editors.
p. ; cm.
Includes bibliographical references and index.
ISBN 978-0-8261-0945-3—ISBN 978-0-8261-0046-0 (e-book) (print)
I. Frith, Karen H. II. Clark, Deborah J. (Deborah Jean), 1958-
[DNLM: 1. Education, Nursing. 2. Education, Distance. 3. Internet. WY 18]
610.73071'1—dc23 2012033581

Printed in the United States of America by Hamilton Printing.

First, I would like to thank Jeanne Novotny for entrusting this work to me. What a gift you gave so freely. I will be a good steward of your original work.

To my husband, Herb, thank you for giving me the space and time to dedicate to my career. Ashley, my daughter, you have brought me joy from the day you were born, and you continue to delight me with your writing and creativity.

To my mother, Ann Harris, you have always believed in me, even when I doubted myself. I knew what a professional woman could achieve because I had the best role model in you. Myra Ashley, my second mother, encouraged me to do what I loved, no matter what the reward. Thank you both for being my cheerleaders.

To my colleagues Jeanne Sewell and Martha Colvin—thank you for instilling the love of educational technology in me and for being my friends. To my mentors Drs. Pamela Levi, Frankie Holder, and Cheryl Kish—I learned about educating nursing students from the best. Thank you for your leadership and for encouraging my scholarship. To my colleagues at UAHuntsville—thanks for making me feel at home and for giving opportunities to grow professionally.

Finally to my students—you keep me on my toes! This book is really about you . . . thinking about how to put you in the center of the teaching–learning experience.

Karen H. Frith

I would like to dedicate this book to my family, friends, colleagues, and students who supported me over the many years of schooling and teaching, day and night, in classrooms and online.

To my husband, Larry Clark, and son, Zachary Clark, who supported my work and school schedules over many years, thank you. I've missed out on a few things while focusing on my career, but you patiently waited. To my mother, Marlene Otto, for encouraging me to continue my studies. To Remy Madison, Molly Sue, and Abraham Lincoln Clark, you bring a smile to my face every time I see you.

To my colleagues and students who stimulated a thirst for innovation and knowledge; you are irreplaceable.

Finally, to my nurse mentors who always thought I could do whatever I set my mind to—Drs. Karen Frith, Alice Demi, and Pamela Levi—you are three very special women!

Deborah J. Clark

Contents

Contributors

Susan Alexander, DNP, RN, CNS, CRNP, BC-ADM Clinical Assistant Professor, College of Nursing, University of Alabama in Huntsville, Huntsville, Alabama

Diane S. Aschenbrenner, MS, RN Instructor, Johns Hopkins University School of Nursing, Baltimore, Maryland

Diane M. Billings, EdD, RN, FAAN Chancellor's Professor Emeritus, Indiana University School of Nursing, Indianapolis, Indiana

Deborah J. Clark, PhD, MSN, MBA, RN, CNE Director, BSN Program, School of Health Science, ECPI University, Virginia Beach, Virginia

Lisa Day, PhD, RN, CNRN Assistant Professor, Duke University School of Nursing, Durham, North Carolina

Suzanne S. Dickerson, DNS, RN Associate Professor and Director of PhD Program, University at Buffalo, State University of New York, Buffalo, New York

Kristina Thomas Dreifuerst, PhD, RN, ACNS-BC, CNE Assistant Professor, Indiana University School of Nursing, Indianapolis, Indiana

Karen H. Frith, PhD, RN, NEA-BC Professor, College of Nursing, University of Alabama in Huntsville, Huntsville, Alabama

Mary J. Greenberg, EdM Project Assistant, PhD Program, University at Buffalo, State University of New York, Buffalo, New York

Desiree Hensel, PhD, RNC-NIC, CNE Assistant Professor, Indiana University, Bloomington, Indiana

Haley Hoy, PhD, ACNP Assistant Professor, College of Nursing, University of Alabama in Huntsville, Huntsville, Alabama

Pamela R. Jeffries, PhD, RN, ANEF, FAAN Associate Dean for Academic Affairs, Johns Hopkins University School of Nursing, Baltimore, Maryland

Arlene E. Johnson, PhD, RN, CPNP Associate Professor, Clemson University School of Nursing, Clemson, South Carolina

Chris Keenan, MSN, RN, CCRN Senior Education Coordinator, SiTEL's Clinical Simulation Centers at MedStar Health, Arlington, Virginia

Marilyn M. Lombardi, PhD Director of Academic and Strategic Technology, Duke University School of Nursing, Durham, North Carolina

Nancy K. Meehan, PhD, RN Associate Professor, Clemson University School of Nursing, Clemson, South Carolina

Marilyn H. Oermann, PhD, RN, ANEF, FAAN Frances Hill Fox Term Distinguished Professor, School of Nursing, University of North Carolina at Chapel Hill, Chapel Hill, North Carolina

Jeanne P. Sewell, MSN, RN-BC Assistant Professor, School of Nursing, Georgia College & State University, Milledgeville, Georgia

Molly Sutphen, PhD Assistant Adjunct Professor, School of Nursing, University of California at San Francisco, San Francisco, California

Brenda S. Talley, PhD, RN, NEA-BC Associate Professor, University of Alabama in Huntsville, Huntsville, Alabama

Joyce B. Vazzano, MS, RN, CRNP Instructor, Johns Hopkins University School of Nursing, Baltimore, Maryland

Bill Wu Yow-Wu, PhD Associate Professor, University at Buffalo, State University of New York, Buffalo, New York

Foreword

Writing a book on distance education in nursing is a difficult and challenging task. Writing any book is difficult, but writing a book on a topic that is changing daily is essentially a never-ending journey and a continuous work in progress. This third edition of *Distance Education in Nursing* is intended for every nurse interested in where we are today in this amazing journey into the future. It addresses issues that cut across a wide range of best practices and the effect of technology on learning. In addition, it gives basic information for those who are thinking about applying some part of technology to their educational, clinical, and research endeavors.

Degree-granting institutions and continuing education programs are facing critical challenges. It is important to understand these challenges. Educational programs must be able to provide quality instruction in rapidly developing areas of knowledge and specialization, meet the learning needs of an increasingly diverse student population, hire faculty that are flexible and have the ability to incorporate research findings and technology into everyday instructional practices, and ensure quality learning standards and professional accreditation criteria. Technology is making it not only possible but also necessary to build evidence in practice that clinical work is truly making a difference in the lives of those we serve. Because of these factors, new ways of addressing the way we teach and how we learn are vitally important.

Although nursing today remains rooted in traditional curriculum models, we are embracing technology as part of mainstream education with new methods of curriculum design and delivery. Technology gives us ever-expanding choices that encourage life-long learning. Also, academic rigor is maintained as we have customized education based on student needs, available technology, and institutional resources.

As you read the chapters in this book, you will discover sound principles and new and creative ideas. There are many implications for future research. What can and cannot be taught online? How are faculty best assisted in learning a new role? Who are the students in this geographically and culturally diverse learning community? When and how are the relationships with students and others changing? How can institutions and students bear the costs?

As I have moved into a new chapter in my life, I have turned my original work in the development of this book over to Dr. Karen Frith. I had the distinct honor of meeting Karen online when we were asked to work together on a committee on online education in academic nursing. Actually, Karen and I have never met face to face. I believe that we are a perfect example of how shared interests and ideas can be created in an online format. In our work together, I came to know that Karen is an expert in the use of technology and informatics and is the perfect person to continue this book. Karen combines her educational role with clinical expertise in nursing administration and leadership, cardiovascular nursing, and nursing research. She has written numerous publications and has been an invited to speak at national and international conferences.

Dr. Deborah Clark is the co-editor of this book and long-time colleague of Karen. She brings not only expertise in online teaching and learning practices to the book, but also administrative experience from serving as the director of an online BSN program and an NLNAC accreditation site visitor. Deborah has examined online experiences of college students and older adults, which gives her a unique perspective about the needs of online learners.

I know that you will enjoy this book because it combines current practices and research with building a foundation of knowledge that takes us into the future. With Karen and Deborah at the helm, the book reflects the best thinking on the state of the art of technology and contemporary leadership.

Jeanne M. Novotny, PhD, RN, FAAN
Dean, School of Nursing
Fairfield University
Fairfield, Connecticut

Preface

In this third edition of *Distance Education in Nursing*, we expand the content and evidence-based practice from the prior edition to represent the explosion of distance teaching and learning over the past several years. Nurse educators are taking advantage of distance learning technologies to make higher education more accessible to potential students and to meet the needs of undergraduate and graduate students in terms of flexibility and learning preferences. Nursing education programs at all levels are incorporating wired and wireless opportunities in traditional classrooms and online. This text is aimed at helping nurse educators of the 21st century in understanding and applying the theoretical bases for distance teaching and learning, while remaining open and interested in cutting-edge technologies. Current educators, new nursing faculty, and students studying nursing education will all benefit from reading this text and applying the concepts to their teaching practices.

There are major differences between the third and second editions. The former edition's chapters retained here (Chapters 2, 3, 5, and 7) have been updated and expanded. New chapters include the first chapter, "Educating Nurses," by Marilyn Lombardi, Molly Sutphen, and Lisa Day. This chapter ties the call for transformation in nursing education to distance education for nursing students. Nurse educators must mindfully design courses and facilitate learning by employing the recommended paradigm shifts. Specific suggestions for overcoming barriers to the paradigm shifts in nursing education, particularly online classes, are discussed in this first chapter.

New chapters on exemplars of faculty preparation (Chapter 4) and student support (Chapter 6) illustrate the journeys of real-life nurse educators in designing, implementing, and evaluating distance education courses and programs, and becoming an expert nurse educator using distance modalities. Their challenges and accomplishments were many and demonstrate the concepts discussed in Chapters 3 and 5. For novice educators, reading the words of these nurses should inspire an appreciation to challenge oneself and continue life-long learning in nursing education.

Leading nurse educators contributed to this text and expanded the discussion on learning objects (Sewell), clinical reasoning and judgment (Jeffries et al.), writing in online education (Oermann), and faculty preparation (Johnson and Meehan). For those considering quality and accreditation needs, Chapter 11 (Billings et al.) answers questions and expands knowledge on measuring quality in distance education and the many challenges of accreditation and regulation. Finally, the last chapter, "There's an App for That!," wraps up current knowledge in wireless and mobile computing for nursing students and educators. Our hope is to continue the community of learning started with this text within the international nurse educator community using a blog and website that will disseminate new evidence-based practice in distance education; new apps and technologies; and shared stories of nurses becoming educators in this wireless world.

Follow our blog at deinnursing.blogspot.com.

Acknowledgments

Distance Education in Nursing, Third Edition, was made possible because of the work of nurse educators from the previous editions and the current edition. We appreciate their contribution to the development of distance education scholarship.

E. Faye Anderson
Diane M. Billings
Tracy Bushee
Suzanne Hetzel Campbell
Cecilia Campos
John M. Clochesy
Karen L. Cobb
Cornelia A. Corbett
Flor Culpa-Bondal
Robert H. Davis
Judith A. Effken
Eunice K. Ernst
Leeann Field
Robert Gibson
Nancy Holloway
Marcella T. Hovancsek
Christine Hudak
Sarah A. Hutchinson
Sonia Jaimovich
Pamela R. Jeffries
Arlene E. Johnson
Stefanie J. Kelly
Joan E. King
Crystal Lane-Tillerson
Ilta Lange
Haeok Lee
Judith M. Lewis
Joan K. Maglivy
Mary L. McHugh
Shirley M. Moore
Carla L. Mueller
Jerry Murley
Julie C. Novak
Jeanne M. Novotny
Susan M. O'Brien
Marilyn H. Oermann
Mary Ann Parsons
Sandra W. Pepicello
Vera Polyakova-Norwood
Linda Royer
Susan D. Schaffer
Marlaine C. Smith
Susan E. Stone
Judith Sweeney
Lucille L. Travis
Mila Urrautia
Patricia Hinton Walker
Tami H. Wyatt
JoAnn Zerwekh

ONE

Educating Nurses
The Call for Transformation of Nursing Education

MARILYN M. LOMBARDI, MOLLY SUTPHEN, and LISA DAY

Nursing education is at a crossroads. With the recent publication of the Carnegie National Study of Nursing Education (Carnegie Foundation for the Advancement of Teaching, 2010) and the Institute of Medicine's (2011) report on the future of nursing, a growing number of nurse educators are questioning whether the models of teaching and learning that currently predominate are sufficient to accomplish the complex, layered, and intellectually challenging learning for practice that student nurses require. For example, in the Carnegie National Study of Nursing Education, Benner, Sutphen, Leonard, and Day (2010) found that the breadth and depth of classroom teaching are weak and that students receive too little help in integrating what they learn in the classroom, the skills lab, and clinical settings. Too often, faculty members in the classroom and clinical setting teach as though they inhabit parallel and separate spheres.

Yet nursing practice requires that students pull together and integrate what they learn in different domains. The domains essential to learning the practice of nursing fall into three general areas of teaching and learning, or what Benner et al. (2010) term *apprenticeships*. In one domain, students learn the knowledge they need for nursing, including knowledge from nursing science, natural sciences, humanities, and social sciences. In another, the apprenticeship of skilled know-how and clinical reasoning, students learn to reason across time about changes in a patient's trajectory as well as the skilled know-how they need to act.

In the third domain, they learn the values, behaviors, standards, social roles, fundamental purposes, and responsibilities that are highly respected in nursing. Benner et al. (2010) refer to these as apprenticeships of knowledge, clinical judgment, and ethical comportment.

The authors of the Carnegie study found a predictable distribution of these three apprenticeships, with knowledge taught in the classroom and skilled know-how taught in the skills/simulation laboratory and clinical settings. Often, the only place where students were consistently asked to learn and integrate their abilities in all three apprenticeships was in the clinical practice setting. The authors call for a radical transformation in how nurses are prepared for practice. To fundamentally transform nursing education, nurse educators must commit to important changes in teaching strategies and pedagogies. Such changes will require considerable commitment on the part of the nursing community including nurses, nursing administrators, faculty, preceptors, and students (Benner et al., 2010). These changes will require all involved to shift approaches, attitudes, assumptions, and goals for nursing education. To this end, Benner et al. (2010) recommend that nurse educators make four fundamental shifts in teaching and learning practices:

1. From a focus on covering decontextualized knowledge to an emphasis on teaching for a sense of salience, situated cognition, and action in particular clinical situations
2. From a sharp separation of clinical and classroom teaching to integration of classroom and clinical teaching
3. From an emphasis on critical thinking to an emphasis on clinical reasoning and multiple ways of thinking that include critical thinking
4. From an emphasis on socialization and role-taking to an emphasis on formation

The focus of this chapter is the four paradigm shifts needed to transform nursing education, the barriers nurse educators face, and the boundaries they must cross in order to make the changes. Then, using each of the paradigm shifts, the current state of the art in distance learning technologies and future education technologies are discussed as they relate to helping teachers overcome barriers and work across boundaries to begin the radical transformation needed in nursing education.

RECOMMENDED "SHIFTS" FROM THE CARNEGIE NATIONAL STUDY OF NURSING EDUCATION

From a Focus on Covering Decontextualized Knowledge to an Emphasis on Teaching for a Sense of Salience, Situated Cognition, and Action in Particular Clinical Situations

Currently, a ubiquitous strategy for presenting nursing theories and clinical knowledge is to provide students with a taxonomy—a classification system of signs, symptoms, and nursing diagnoses related to specific diseases. A taxonomy may be useful for organizing large amounts of information, but few students can figure out how isolated facts presented in lectures are supposed to be used in particular situations when caring for patients whose needs may not fit neatly into such a classification system.

Students need help in learning how to use the nursing knowledge and science presented in lectures, during simulations, and in the clinical setting. Part of learning a practice is developing a sense of salience or a sense of what is important in complex, relatively unstructured clinical situations in which patient care takes place. To act, nurses must learn to grasp the nature of the situation and be able to distinguish what nursing care is needed. Students develop a sense of salience through ongoing coaching, where preceptors, faculty, and nurses coach students through questions about particular situations and the changing relevance, demands, resources, and constraints they encounter.

From a Sharp Separation of Clinical and Classroom Teaching to Integration of Classroom and Clinical Teaching

Currently, student nurses experience a sharp divide between classroom and clinical teaching and learning. Such a structural separation of clinical settings from the classroom often means students are left on their own to integrate what they learn in each setting. Students, however, need help with the integration of clinical and classroom teaching and learning. By integrating clinical and classroom learning into a seamless whole, nurse educators could prevent the fragmentation students currently experience. This integration would also potentially take some of the burden of content overload off teachers and students by limiting the discussion to the concerns and problems of actual clients/patients and communities. Better integration can be accomplished by bringing clinical situations into the classroom and lab with simulation and case studies, by bringing classroom learning and assignments into clinical settings, and by involving faculty in all teaching/learning settings.

From an Emphasis on Critical Thinking to an Emphasis on Clinical Reasoning and Multiple Ways of Thinking That Include Critical Thinking

Currently, "critical thinking" has become the catchall phrase to describe how nurses think in practice, and many teachers and students believe that critical thinking is the only way nurses think. However, the term does not begin to capture the many ways nurses think—creatively, analytically, imaginatively, and narratively, for example. Although student nurses must be able to use critical thinking, they also need to be able to distinguish when and why this kind of thinking is required. Critical thinking is important in situations of practice breakdown or if a situation prompts reflection on outmoded theories, received ideas, and practices that need reform or innovation.

In order for student nurses to learn and practice all the different kinds of thinking that make up clinical reasoning and judgment, nurse educators must be more direct in the ways they talk about their own thinking and more explicit in how they teach students how to think like nurses. Much of nursing practice requires action in underdetermined situations where there is neither sufficient information nor time to critically think through every possibility. Through careful coaching in particular clinical situations, nurses, faculty, and clinical preceptors help students learn the different ways of thinking nurses use and help students develop a clinical imagination to see possibilities, resources, and constraints in patient and family situations that demand action. Especially effective are "what-if" questions posed by faculty about a particular clinical situation that ask students to grasp the nature of patients' needs as they change over time. Likewise, helping students develop a narrative understanding and interpretation of clinical situations can enrich clinical imagination and reasoning about changes in the patient's condition over time.

From an Emphasis on Socialization and Role-Taking to an Emphasis on Formation

Student nurses describe their work with clients, patients, and families as transformative of how they see the larger world, their future, and themselves. Despite the students' experiences of transformation, formation in nursing education is often overlooked in favor of discussions of role transition. Foster, Dahill, Golemon, and Tolentino (2006) define formation as the pedagogies used by educators to form in students the ". . . dispositions, habits, knowledge, and skills that cohere in professional identity and practice, commitments and integrity" (p. 100). In this sense, the formation of new nurses is closely tied to their internal identification with the values of nursing practice and is different from socialization into a role. When one is socialized or takes on a role, expectations are externally imposed, and good performance is demonstrated by acting in accordance with a set of externally defined criteria. As such, it is assumed one can put on the role of nurse when it is needed and other times step out of this role. In contrast, when the values of a practice are internalized, new nurses develop an inner sense of good that influences their judgment of right and wrong action in all situations. Educating nurses as professionals with a commitment to service and advocacy requires attending overtly and deliberately to formation in the curriculum and in teaching and learning.

BARRIERS TO ACCOMPLISHING THE FOUR PARADIGM SHIFTS

In the past, there have been many calls for reform in nursing education from curriculum reform to pedagogical innovation (National League for Nursing, 2003). There are many reasons why reform efforts have been neither widespread nor lasting. In order to accomplish the transformation called for by the authors of the Carnegie study, it will be important to identify barriers to change within teachers, students, and schools. Such barriers include the overwhelming amount of content teachers and students feel compelled to address in classroom teaching and learning, the absence of generalist knowledge among nursing faculty, and the hierarchical relationships that have been established between teachers and students.

The information explosion in health care is overwhelming to many nurses, nurse educators, and student nurses (Benner et al., 2010). Medical–surgical nursing textbooks are now multivolume tomes with an accompanying CD-ROM and website. The Internet is a sea of clinical practice guidelines and websites for health care providers and the general public, providing information on wellness, illness, and diseases. In sorting through all of this content, many nurse educators are most comfortable constructing a slide-based lecture followed by multiple-choice tests to assess student learning. Teachers who may have limited teaching skills and feel pressured to cover large amounts of content often rely exclusively on lecture; students come to expect this format and get nervous when there is a change. Likewise, school administrators are fearful that without lecture and multiple-choice exams, students will not be prepared adequately for the national licensing exam (NCLEX-RN®). Thus, reliance on lecture and on multiple-choice testing acts as a barrier to improvement in teaching and learning.

Another important barrier occurs when the teacher overlooks the type of practice that a novice could enter. Because there is a division of classroom and clinical teaching/learning in many schools of nursing, the teachers in the classroom often do not have any connection to the clinical sites where students practice. In addition, many faculty members are experts in a particular clinical practice but lack the generalist knowledge required to cross clinical specialties even within a larger specialty. For example, a cardiovascular nurse practitioner who is teaching a class on acute care of adults may be comfortable covering the content associated with cardiac disease but not with neuroscience. For topics outside of the specialty, nurse educators typically use taxonomies of signs, symptoms, and treatments, rather than teaching with rich case studies derived from their clinical experience. This specialty clinical practice makes it difficult for teachers to move away from classroom teaching that relies on classifications of diseases and treatment options.

Another important barrier to making the paradigm shifts is the hierarchy in place in many schools, with teacher as knowledge-giving expert and students as empty receptacles. Moving from a programmed lecture to a less predictable learning environment where students and teacher work together to think about and respond to contextualized clinical problems will require a different understanding of and approach to student–teacher relationships. In the current model in place in many nursing schools, the classroom teacher is responsible for filling the students up with the content they need for practice; the students are expected to then take this content and apply it in their clinical settings. This passive learning environment reinforces a separation of teacher and student, encourages competition among students, and prevents more collaborative relationships from forming.

BOUNDARIES ON THE WAY TO TRANSFORMATION

In moving toward integration of the three apprenticeships of professional education in nursing, faculties in schools of nursing will have to make conscious efforts to dismantle three closely related boundaries: the boundary between theory and practice, the boundary between knowledge acquisition and knowledge use, and the boundary between classroom and clinical learning. Breaking through these boundaries is implied in the paradigm shifts that address the separation of knowledge from context and the separation of classroom from clinical learning. However, overcoming these boundaries will also bring nursing education closer to the shift from critical thinking to multiple modes of thinking and from socialization to formation.

The favoring of theory over practice and of knowing over doing is an old problem in Western science (Benner, 1984; Benner, Tanner, & Chesla, 1996). While acknowledging the importance of hands-on skills, it is still a common understanding among nurse educators that students must learn the theory before they can apply it in practice and that a solid theoretical understanding should result in solid clinical practice. However, in nursing, the practice is always more complex, flexible, and responsive than a theory can capture, and the ability to use knowledge in undetermined and changing situations is essential (Benner, 1984; Benner et al., 1996; Benner, Hooper-Kyriakidis, & Stannard, 1999). By creating learning environments that recognize practice as an important source of knowledge and theory and engagement with a community of practice as the basic source of learning (Lave & Wenger, 1991), nurse educators will be able to cross the boundary between theory and practice and close the practice–education gap.

Closely related to the theory–practice boundary is the boundary between knowledge acquisition and knowledge use. Learning science tells us that students learn best by using knowledge as they acquire it (Chickering & Gamson, 1987; Tokuhama-Espinosa, 2010). Nursing schools must become places where students are always asked to confront clinical problems that require them to learn and use new content. This blending of knowledge acquisition and knowledge use also will help students better understand the demands of the practice they are entering and further their professional formation.

In essence, dismantling the boundaries between theory and practice, knowledge acquisition and knowledge use, begins with an effort to identify the most valuable features of the clinical placement experience and transport those features, as far as possible, beyond the clinical setting into the classroom and the online realm. Simply put, the clinical setting is the one learning environment where students are asked to bring together the four fundamental "patterns of knowing" that underlie professional practice in nursing as identified by Barbara Carper (1978) in her well-known formulation: empirical, personal, ethical, and aesthetic (as in, related to the here and now). Carper's vision of an expert nurse is one who is able to integrate these patterns of knowing when it counts the most. However, in order to do so, expert nurses must engage in a process of lifelong learning known as *reflective practice*. Thus, when faced with a clinical issue, these nurses are able to think on their feet, but they also take the time to document their reaction to the situation after the fact and reflect on the consequences of their actions. Over time, this reflective practice hones the professional's sense of salience or the ability to prioritize in a complex, ambiguous clinical situation and immediately determine what needs to be attended to before anything else.

TRANSFORMATION OF NURSING IN DISTANCE EDUCATION

In many ways, the transformation of nursing education described by Benner et al. (2010) is already taking place in distance education. Dedicated nurse educators faced with moving courses from face-to-face classrooms into online, virtual classrooms quickly realized that simply putting lectures online would fail. The pioneers of online education made a monumental shift from teacher-centered pedagogy to leaner-centered pedagogy. Some authors even extol the learner-centered practices of distance education as having a positive influence on classroom teaching practices (Shovein, Huston, Fox, & Damazo, 2005; Stone & Perumean-Chaney, 2011).

The learner-centered pedagogy of distance education that predominates leans heavily on educational theories such as constructivism and adult learning theory. Both of these purport that learning occurs best when it is situated in meaningful contexts; when learners can connect new ideas to their previous knowledge, experience, or emotions; and when the learning is authentic or based in real situations. Because adult learners tend to value previous experience, self-directed reflective practice, and creative problem solving in dialogue with others, they also tend to respond positively to constructivist learning activities (Lombardi, 2007). Nurse educators who design instruction will likely use learning management systems that contain technology able to shift the educational paradigm. However, the transformation will require a purposeful and creative instructional design.

While nursing faculty rarely have formal training in pedagogy, they are quite skilled in developing learning objectives in courses that support program objectives. When developing or redesigning distance education courses with transformation in mind, the same principles are used—imagine the knowledge, skills, and values of students that are desired, and create structures and processes to support the desired outcomes.

Each technology is a tool with its own set of affordances, or the *range of possibilities* that opens up for the user, and its own set of constraints, or the range of possibilities that this technology closes off for the user. Once educators clarify the learning context (characteristics of learners, student level, the nature of the learning environment, etc.) and learning intent (what the student will be required to do/demonstrate/produce at the conclusion of the lesson/module/unit), they are ready to determine which technologies are best suited to serving the educational purpose, given the particular learning context and intent.

Fortunately, there are a number of models available to help instructors match learning intent with learning strategies, and strategies with technology supports. One such model identified five fundamental learning intents and produced the following matrix (Table 1.1; Littlejohn & Pegler, 2007).

Those who teach at an institution with a robust distance education program can expect to have at their disposal an infrastructure that includes high-speed Internet connectivity, access to mobile and stationary computing devices, systems for producing and presenting multimedia materials and capturing information about student performance by way of learning management systems, asynchronous and synchronous communication, and social networking tools for the support of teamwork and peer-based learning. Nurse educators must select carefully the instructional technologies amid a vast and rapidly changing digital world. Each instructional design decision has the opportunity to overcome barriers and push traditional boundaries in the goal of transforming nursing education.

Paradigms 1 and 2: Teaching for a Sense of Salience, Situated Cognition, and Action in Particular Situations and Integrating Classroom and Clinical Teaching

One of the most effective ways of teaching for a sense of salience and collapsing the distance between the clinical setting and the classroom (or clinical and the virtual learning environment) is a pedagogy built on unfolding case studies. Many case studies are available from online repositories or websites dedicated to online delivery of cases. The National Center for Case Study Teaching in Science (2012) contains a collection of unfolding cases in nursing and many other science disciplines. The site also provides learning objectives and teaching suggestions for in-class collaborative learning, but the ideas are easily transferable to online collaborative case studies. Other free sources of case studies can be found in the Multimedia Educational Resource for Learning and Online Teaching (MERLOT, 2012). Educators in all disciplines have

TABLE 1.1 Learning Intents and Section of Instructional Technologies

Learning Intent	What Is It?	Media Forms	Active-Learning Strategies	Support Tools
Assimilative	Students are asked to process narrative media while managing and structuring information	Content delivery in multimedia formats (readings, lectures, narrated slide presentations, etc.)	Web quests, concept mapping, mind mapping, brainstorming, participatory sense making	Learning management systems (Blackboard, Sakai, Moodle, etc.), presentation software, brainstorming tools including concept mapping software, citation/research management tools including social bookmarking software, news aggregators (e.g., Google Reader), reflective journaling software (blogs), and collaboration software (wikis that support group work, including multiauthor annotated bibliographies)
Adaptive	An environment that changes according to learner input	Clinical simulations, game-based assessment environments	Situated coaching through online learning and assessment modules	Task-centered online learning modules (including a series of questions, decision points, and requests for rationale that students must address), role-playing exercises performed in multiplayer online role-playing game environments, interactive web-based lessons and clinical cases like NovEx eLearning
Communicative	Discussing	Asynchronous or synchronous discussions, chats, text messages	Reasoning, arguing, coaching, debate, discussion, negotiation, performance, online peer critique	Electronic whiteboards, e-mail, discussion boards, chat, instant messaging, VoIP (Voice over Internet Protocol, i.e., Internet telephony applications such as Skype), video conferencing, blogs, wikis
Productive	Learners producing something	Creating, producing, writing, synthesizing, remixing, mash-ups	Patient care plan, reflective journal, literature review, portfolio, narrated slide presentation	Creative applications (Google Video, office software, InDesign, Photoshop, Sketch, and other design software), publishing environments (YouTube), computer-aided assessment tools, electronic learning environments
Experiential	Interactive activities that focus on problem solving in a variety of clinical situations	Practicing, applying, mimicking, experiencing, exploring, investigating, performing	Case studies, simulation scenarios, role-playing exercises, interprofessional team-based learning	Multimedia, interactive case study lessons (NovEx eLearning), virtual simulation labs that approximate clinical settings and conditions within a 3-D immersive environment, massively multiplayer online role-playing games

contributed nearly 31,000 learning objects (materials or assessments in self-contained modules that can be reused). Textbook publishers and other commercial websites offer case studies that can be integrated into online classes such as Evolve and Lippincott's multimedia packages. Access to learning materials tends to be similar to the cost of textbooks.

A new online learning system based on the "novice-to-expert learning" approach is being pioneered by Benner (NovEx Novice to Expert Learning®, 2011). Launched in response to the call for an increase in situated (context-specific) learning issued by the Carnegie Foundation, the Robert Wood Johnson Foundation, the Institute of Medicine, Quality & Safety Education for Nurses (2011), and the Lancet Commission (Frenk et al., 2010), the NovEx eLearning system comprises a growing set of online courses that instructors are encouraged to use as a replacement for the traditional textbook. Students access a set of online modules that include short digital lessons focused on essential clinical and scientific information, along with videos that visually reinforce proper clinical use of concepts under discussion. Students immediately use the knowledge learned from the NovEx lessons by practicing on "unfolding" patient cases designed by content experts to reflect the latest evidence-based practices. An example of curatorial teaching, the NovEx case approach displays important artifacts (the patient in the clinical context, medical images, video interviews, electronic medical records, instrument readouts, etc.) in a sequence designed to create a pathway through the unfolding situation with students called upon to use all four patterns of knowing fundamental to a nurse's reflective practice. Students may repeat the interactive tutorial as often as they wish and receive feedback on their performances. Finally, they are prepared to enter the online test "rooms" where interaction with the clinical situation is tracked and assessed. Significantly, there is a transformative agenda behind this new e-learning program, which presents nurse educators with templates and guidelines they can follow in crafting their own unfolding case study scenarios. In this way, the online tutorials help to shift nursing education away from decontextualized lectures and toward a context-based pedagogy that engages students in meaningful dialogue.

Paradigm 3: Emphasis on Clinical Reasoning and Multiple Ways of Thinking

Authentic learning experiences are designed to evoke, as closely as possible, the complex, open-ended dynamics found in actual practice, where problems typically require input from multiple perspectives. As learning scientist George Siemens (2004) suggests, learning to be a professional nurse is all about forging connections—interpersonal connections between mentors and learners, intellectual connections between the familiar and the novel, private connections between the individual learner's goals and the broader concerns of the discipline. It is through the many and varied exposures that students begin to think deeper and broader about situations in patient care. Differences in perspectives, similarity of human needs, and scientific thinking are enhanced when students are challenged to solve problems and reflect on practice.

Online discussions can be used to enhance clinical reasoning; an introductory topic is posted for discussion, and student response is based on readings. Faculty take the topic to the next level by posting intriguing, thought-provoking responses and additional questions that stimulate students to use their clinical reasoning and critical thinking abilities. It is the creative online educator that can develop discussion topics that are relevant and intriguing enough to push students to use their higher-level thinking abilities, combined with practice experience, to find solutions to practice issues.

Paradigm 4: Emphasis on Formation

Finally, it is imperative for student nurses to become lifelong learners responsible for their own growth and responsiveness as clinicians. As educational theorist Gardner Campbell (2009) insisted, students must acquire the "digital fluency" necessary for them to assume "creative and responsible leadership." Nurse educators can mentor students in formation as professional nurses and lifelong learners using online tools that engage them, foster inquiry, and create opportunities for robust discussion. In a networked, technology-enriched world, the educator can bring quality content to students and create a pathway through the content that fosters reflection *in* action and reflection *on* action. Narrative pedagogies lend support to other forms of generative sharing, including "digital stories" culled from previous experiences related to the topic at hand. Students might be asked to contribute to the curated resources by using a simple tool such as VoiceThread™ (2012) to combine images and words into a 3- to 5-minute video that others in the class may comment on with the help of VoiceThread's annotation tool.

As an adult learning community, students in a well-developed online course will work together to reflect on their past and current experiences to create materials that demonstrate their ability to "think like a nurse." The artifacts they produce over the course, in the form of patient care plans, for instance, should ultimately contribute to the learning community's shared base of resources that have been vetted for their reliability and usefulness. The longevity of these resources and the learning community building around them can be assured through the use of electronic portfolios that help students see the arc of their progress over time or collaborative wikis where members of the learning community can work jointly to develop a common knowledge base. The nurse educator models the curatorial behavior of the lifelong learner by designing a pathway through the content.

Before they graduate, student nurses should be able to create and maintain a *personal learning network* that will support their lifelong learning needs. They can join professional communities and reach out electronically to potential mentors. They should be exposed to social bookmarking tools and academic reference management systems (e.g., Mendeley, Zotero, Endnote) that allow them to work together with nurses from across the country and around the world to construct online collections of Internet resources or bookmarks, classify and organize them through the use of metadata tags, and share both the bookmarks and tags with others. As professional nurses, they have an obligation to keep up to date on significant changes in the field as efficiently as possible by subscribing to the syndicated Web content (news headlines, podcasts, blogs, etc.) published by significant organizations and thought leaders in their field. Aggregator tools (or "news readers") will automatically assemble that syndicated Web content into a "personal newspaper" dedicated to the user's particular interests and affinities. Even though these are digital skills, student nurses who learn to harness digital resources also are forming into lifelong learners.

SUMMARY AND KEY POINTS

Nurse educators who prepare students for entry-level or advanced nursing practice have the responsibility of designing instruction that captures the realities of fast-paced and uncertain work environments. Using instruction that calls on clinical imagination and thinking in context can be achieved in online education. The role of the nurse educator is to serve as coach and guide through learner-centered online education.

Key Points

1. The call for radical transformation of nursing education is important for teachers in distance education. It is the role of every nurse educator to design distance education courses that shift from traditional teaching methods to those that encourage students to think as nurses.
2. Transformation of nursing education means that teachers move from presenting information to guiding students to understand the most significant clinical issues and using knowledge in context. Teachers in online courses can use many different instructional technology tools to situate learning in context, including case studies and simulations.
3. Transformation means that nurse educators close the gap between classroom and clinical settings. By using case studies and other clinically realistic multimedia learning objects, nurse educators are able to showcase clinical learning even in online courses.
4. Nurse educators will transform education when they encourage students to develop clinical reasoning and to use multiple ways of thinking. In distance education, self-reflection in blogs, group collaboration in wikis, and thought-provoking online discussions can promote deep thinking and sharing of ideas with peers.
5. The final paradigm shift involves moving from socialization to an emphasis on formation in nursing education. Formation is a process of internalizing the values of nursing practice. Nurse educators play a vital role in developing an online community of learners who appreciate responsibilities for evidence-based, ethical practice.

REFERENCES

Benner, P. (1984). *From novice to expert: Excellence and power in clinical nursing practice.* Menlo Park, CA: Addison-Wessley.

Benner, P., Tanner, C., & Chesla, C. (1996). *Expertise in nursing practice: Caring, clinical judgment and ethics.* New York, NY: Springer.

Benner, P., Hooper-Kyriakidis, P., & Stannard, D. (1999). *Clinical wisdom and interventions in critical care: A thinking-in-action approach.* Philadelphia, PA: Saunders.

Benner, P., Sutphen, M., Leonard, V., & Day, L. (2010). *Educating nurses: A call for radical transformation.* San Francisco, CA: Jossey-Bass. Retrieved from http://www.carnegiefoundation.org/publications/educating-nurses-call-radical-transformation

Campbell, G. (2009). A personal cyberinfrastructure. *EDUCAUSE Review, 44*(5), 58–59.

Carnegie Foundation for the Advancement of Teaching. (2010). *Carnegie calls for 'radical transformation' of nursing education.* Retrieved from http://www.carnegiefounda

tion.org/carnegie-perspectives/carnegie-calls-%E2%80%98radical-transformation%E2%80%99-nursing-education

Carper, B. (1978). Fundamental patterns of knowing in nursing. *Advances in Nursing Science, 1*(1): 13–23.

Chickering, A. W., & Gamson, Z. F. (1987). Seven principles for good practice in undergraduate education. *American Association for Higher Education Bulletin, 39,* 3–7.

Foster, C. R., Dahill, L. E., Golemon, L. A., & Tolentino, B. W. (2006). *Educating clergy: Teaching practices and pastoral imagination.* San Francisco, CA: Jossey-Bass.

Frenk, J., Chen, L., Bhutta, Z. A., Cohen, J., Crisp, N., Evans, T. ...Zurayk, H. (2010). Health professionals for a new century: Transforming education to strengthen health systems in an interdependent world. *The Lancet, 376*(9756), 1923–1958.

Institute of Medicine. Committee on the Robert Wood Johnson Foundation Initiative on the Future of Nursing. (2011). *The future of nursing: Leading change, advancing health.* Washington, DC: The National Academies Press. Retrieved from http://books.nap.edu/openbook.php?record_id=12956

Lave, J., & Wenger, E. (1991). *Situated learning: Legitimate peripheral participation.* New York, NY: Cambridge University Press.

Littlejohn, A., & Pegler, C. (2007). *Preparing for blended e-learning.* London, England: Routledge.

Lombardi, M. M. (2007). *Authentic learning for the 21st century: An overview. Educause.* Retrieved from http://net.educause.edu/ir/library/pdf/ELI3009.pdf

MERLOT. (2012). Home page. Retrieved from http://www.merlot.org/merlot/index.htm

National Center for Case Study Teaching in Science. (2012). Retrieved from http://sciencecases.lib.buffalo.edu/cs/

National League for Nursing. (2003). Innovation in nursing education: A call to reform. In *NLN Board of Governors Position Statement.* Retrieved from http://www.nln.org/aboutnln/ positionstatements/innovation082203.pdf

NovEx Novice to Expert Learning. (2011). About NovEx. Retrieved from http://novicetoexpert.org/AboutNovEx

Quality & Safety Education for Nurses. (2011). Welcome. Retrieved from http://www.qsen.org/

Shovein, J., Huston, C., Fox, S., & Damazo, B. (2005). Challenging traditional teaching and learning paradigms: Online learning and emancipatory teaching. *Nursing Education Perspectives, 26*(6), 340–343.

Siemens, G. (2004). *Connectivism: A learning theory for the digital age.* Retrieved from http://www.elearnspace.org/Articles/connectivism.htm

Stone, M., & Perumean-Chaney, S. (2011). The benefits of online teaching for traditional classroom pedagogy: A case study for improving face-to-face instruction. *JOLT, 7*(3). Retrieved from http://jolt.merlot.org/vol7no3/stone_0911.htm

Tokuhama-Espinosa, T. (2010). *The new science of teaching and learning: Using the best of mind, brain, and education science in the classroom.* New York, NY: Teacher's College Press.

VoiceThread. (2012). VoiceThread overview. Retrieved from http://voicethread.com/about/features/

TWO

An Overview of Distance Education and Online Courses

KAREN H. FRITH

Ted, a clinical nurse specialist, drives to the campus of the state university. He feels some unease because every time he goes to school, he understands just how much more there is to learn about patient care. This time is different—Ted will be the teacher. Ted learned during the interview that he would be expected to use the Internet to teach campus-based and online classes. Questions run through his head like the playlist on his MP3 device.

- I'm a great nurse, but how can I help others to learn to think like a nurse?
- In my educator role at the hospital, I assisted nurses when they were unsure about their patients. I really liked that part of my job. How can I convey complex patient situations to my students when I teach online?
- When I went to school, our teachers gave lectures, and we took tests. I am expected to teach online—where do I learn how to be a competent teacher using a method I have never experienced?
- I know there are software programs that I can use to develop interesting learning activities. Will I have time to learn everything? Who will help me? How will I know whether or not I'm a good teacher?

Susan finishes her workout at the fitness center before her shift starts in the emergency department. She likes the fast pace of her work and enjoys learning something new every day. It has been 3 years since Susan finished an Associate of Science in Nursing degree (ADN). She has begun to consider returning to college to complete a Bachelor of

Science in Nursing (BSN). The local college is conveniently located 20 minutes from home but offers only day classes that will conflict with her work schedule. She considers online programs because she took Internet-enhanced courses in her ADN program. Susan uses her computer a great deal at work for charting and at home for banking, shopping online, reading news, and talking to friends on Facebook. She finds an assessment tool to check her readiness for learning online. Her score on the assessment shows that she is self-motivated, has good time management skills, and is competent with basic computer activities. After considering her options, Susan decides to enroll in an online BSN program for registered nurses (RN-BSN) program at the state university.

These examples demonstrate how the Internet has revolutionized nursing education. If Ted had started his academic career just 10 years earlier, teaching online would not have been discussed in his interview. Now Ted needs to learn how to teach effectively in the classroom, clinical setting, and online. Susan has opportunities to continue her education because of distance education programs. She gets access to a quality education that fits her schedule. Today, whether students enroll in a traditional campus-based program or learn at a distance, the Internet influences the way they learn.

Online education is gaining traction as a mainstream method for providing postsecondary education. In a report by the National Center for Education Statistics (NCES, 2011), nearly 4.3 million undergraduate students took at least one distance education class. This number represents a 25% increase from the reported number in the academic year 2003–2004. The percentage of students using distance education to complete an entire program is low, with estimates of only 3.7%. However, graduate students comprise a higher percentage than undergraduate students for online program completion (NCES, 2011).

The purposes of this chapter are to introduce key concepts in distance education and to describe the background and relevant issues in distance education. Inherent in these discussions are the advantages and limitations of distance education. Comparisons and contrasts between on-campus education and distance education will be made where appropriate.

KEY CONCEPTS DEFINED

Distance Education

Distance education is defined as planned learning that occurs in a different place from teaching, requiring real-time (synchronous) or delayed (asynchronous) interactive technology and needing a course design supportive of students (Escoffery, Miner, & Alperin, 2003). Holden and Westfall (2006) add that distance education is part of a curriculum in which course objectives provide structure and assessment of learning is measured. The definition of distance education does not include any particular method or medium; rather, it focuses on teaching and learning with technology as a conduit. At the writing of this book, the most common method of providing distance education is based on Internet technologies.

In the following paragraphs, other commonly used terms are defined for the reader. Those wishing to review additional terms can refer to the National Council of State Boards of Nursing (n.d.) at www.ncsbn.org/836.htm and the United States Distance Learning Association (USDLA) at www.usdla.org/distance-learning-glossary (Simonson, 2008).

Traditional Courses and Internet-Supported Courses

In contrast to distance education, traditional on-campus courses are taught in college or university classrooms at least once per week. On-campus courses are also known as *face-to-face (f2f)*, *in-seat*, or *on-site courses*. Teachers in on-campus courses may design courses and their assignments without requiring students to use the Internet. It is likely that most on-campus courses have morphed into Internet-supported (also called web-enhanced) courses, which have credit-hour-driven requirements for in-seat time and have at least some course materials available on the Internet, thus making use of the Internet as a repository (Parsad & Lewis, 2008). Some Internet-supported courses offer additional interaction using e-mail and discussion groups *in a learning management system* (LMS), which is software developed for design, delivery, and management of online classes.

Hybrid Courses

A hybrid course (also called blended course) is a course that has both in-seat and online course requirements. The key to this definition is that there is a reduction in the in-seat time (Parsad & Lewis, 2008). There is no widely accepted definition of the percentage of time for the on-campus and online components, nor is there a set way to arrange the on-campus requirements. For example, some hybrid courses require students to have one or more days of intensive classes on campus followed by some weeks or months of online work. Other hybrid courses alternate weeks for on-campus and online work. Some teachers feel that these hybrid courses overcome the limitations of a fully online course (loss of the face-to-face meetings between instructor and student and loss of demonstrations that teachers believe can be done only in person) but allow people to be distance students because they require fewer days of on-campus work. The limiting factor for students is having sufficient control over their work and family schedules to meet the on-campus requirements.

Online Courses

An *online course* or *e-learning course* is one in which the entire course is offered through the Internet. The syllabus, including course description, objectives, course schedule, handouts, examinations, class discussions, and so on are all available only through the Internet, typically in an LMS. Students must have access to a computer or other electronic device with reliable Internet service. Some courses require special software and hardware in order for students to fully participate. Students typically communicate with each other and with the teacher via a combination of discussion boards, chat rooms, and e-mail. The teacher may or may not provide lecture materials to support required readings. Typically, teachers provide information about important links to relevant sites on the Internet, but students are also expected to do personal searches to enhance their own learning. An online course usually adheres to the traditional semester or quarter schedule of the university in which it is housed.

Some academic programs combine various forms of distance-education modalities to attract students in far-off places. These programs, known as *external degree programs*, use video or film technology, print media, videoconferencing technology, and the Internet to deliver instruction. They differ from other distance education offerings because students typically engage in courses at their own pace, and the start and end dates of the class do not have to fit into the university's usual calendar (unless students are receiving financial aid). Students who enroll in external degree programs learn independently by completing modules or learning contracts, and they have little interaction with other students. Some universities offer external degree programs exclusively and have no campus for classes.

There is no one standard way to offer distance education. Within a college or university, academic departments often have the freedom to choose how much distance education will be used and what type of technology is suitable to meet the demand for programs. For example, a nursing department might use online exclusively, and a department of engineering might distribute digital versatile disks (DVDs) for content and use videoconferencing to interact with students. Even within a department, the extent of distance education can be different—an entire RN-BSN could be online, but prelicensure students enrolled in a BSN program might only have Internet-supported classes.

Not only is the amount of distance education fluid, but also the type of media used changes as technologies improve. It is likely that mobile technology such as smartphones, tablets, and other handheld technology that have the capability to display e-mail, Internet content, and video conferencing will have a prominent role in distance education in the near future (Holden & Westfall, 2010). Immersive environments such as Second Life, OpenSimulator, and Sloodle (combination of Moodle and Second Life) are beginning to be used in distance education, bringing gaming and role-playing into the educational experience (Briggs, 2010). Another potential innovative technology is augmented reality, which provides a way to combine mobile technology with "location awareness." For example, a nurse could use a mobile device in proximity to medical equipment, and a pop-up menu of frequently asked questions for that equipment would appear on the mobile device (Raths, 2012). Distance education is as innovative as the imagination of academic and professional development leaders and educators. Those with vision and a willingness to take risks will define distance education in the future.

Modes of Online Education

The two basic modes of online education are synchronous and asynchronous interaction (Table 2.1). Parsad and Lewis (2008) reported that 75% of degree-granting institutions used asynchronous modes to a large extent in distance education. Asynchronous learning occurs when individuals access the educational materials independently and at times and places of their choice. Asynchronous activities allow students to take as much time as they want to read the materials and compose responses or messages. It also allows time for reflection and may result in thoughtful discussion. The use of asynchronous technology extends the reach of education to previously underserved populations as well as to those who prefer a more self-directed learning environment. It is

TABLE 2.1 Asynchronous Versus Synchronous Distance Learning via the Internet

Learning methodology	Asynchronous	Synchronous
Video	• Prerecorded webinars • Videoconference • Prerecorded lecture	• Real-time videoconference streaming • One-way videoconferencing: Learner can see and hear the conference but cannot interact with the speaker • Two-way videoconferencing: Learner can see, hear, and interact with the speaker by typing responses or by voice and video with videoconferencing technology
Document sharing/ assignments	• Sending documents or assignments via e-mail • "Cloud" storage of documents such as Google Docs	• Sharing of documents using courseware management systems or other applications that allow real-time document sharing
Discussion	• Listservs • Threaded discussions • Newsgroups • E-mail • Social media • Immersive environments	• Chat rooms • Real-time videoconferencing • Immersive environments
Presentations	• Multimedia or electronic presentations • Case studies • Video tutorials • Webcasts • Text-based tutorials • Interactive tutorials	• Real-time videoconference streaming • Audio/document sharing
Evaluation	• Online surveys • Tests • Threaded discussions • Newsgroups • Listservs • Document sharing	• Real-time document • Audio sharing • Videoconference streaming

the most flexible and friendly way to use the Internet for formal degree programs and continuing education. Although not used as frequently, synchronous modes allow the teacher and students to interact in real time, similar to traditional classroom settings. This method decreases flexibility by requiring all students to be online, in a videoconference, or in a virtual classroom at the same time.

ONLINE LEARNING IS A WIN FOR HIGHER EDUCATION

Using computer technology and the Internet has soared to the forefront of distance education partly because of technological advances that are available on college campuses and in homes of potential students, and partly because online education is seen as way to attract and retain students (Allen & Seaman, 2011). Increased enrollment in online courses filled some of the funding gaps in higher education that resulted from the economic downturn in the late 2000s. (Instructional Technology Council, 2011). The decision to offer online classes has paid off—the growth rate of U.S. students taking online courses has exceeded the growth rate of all students in higher education in the United States (Allen & Seaman, 2011). In response to the bigger role that teaching online is playing in higher education, the *U.S. News & World Report* (Sheehy, 2012) annually ranks online bachelor's programs. The ranking criteria are focused on three critical areas: faculty credentials and training, student services and technology, and student engagement and assessment. These areas will be addressed in part in this and subsequent chapters.

Degree-granting institutions are facing critical challenges because nurses entering health care careers will experience rapidly changing demands for knowledge and skills. In order to remain competitive, institutions of higher education and nursing programs must do the following:

- Provide first-rate leadership with clear vision in rapidly developing, new areas of knowledge and specialization (Institute of Medicine, 2011)
- Create opportunities for seamless progression from one degree program to the next higher level (Institute of Medicine, 2011)
- Hire faculty who are flexible and have the ability to incorporate research findings and technology into everyday instructional practices (Johnson, Smith, Willis, Levine, & Haywood, 2011)
- Provide professional development to ensure all faculty are competent with instructional technologies, particularly online learning (Paulus et al., 2010)
- Create an environment supportive of innovation in teaching and learning practices (Benner, Sutphen, Leonard, & Day, 2010)
- Meet the learning needs of an increasingly diverse student population (Marcyjanik & Zom, 2011)
- Ensure quality learning standards and accreditation criteria that are comparable to face-to-face formats (Commission on Collegiate Nursing Education, 2009; National League for Nursing Accreditation Commission, 2008)

Because of these challenges, new ways of addressing teaching and learning are of the utmost importance. As universities, associations, private providers, and others compete in the marketplace for formal and continuing professional education, increasing numbers of learners will turn to the Internet as a convenient, satisfying, and economically prudent way to save time and money in order to keep current in their field.

Advantages of Online Learning

Distance education offers new opportunities for nurses who are seeking basic or advanced degrees, certificates, or lifelong learning for professional development. The advantages to using the Internet are many. Online education is an important avenue of learning for practicing nurses and nursing students who live busy lives and who have great difficulty with scheduling. Nurses work different shifts—scheduling 3 or 4 hours a week in class at the same time every week for 15 weeks may be impossible. The ability of students to participate in class and do assignments at their own convenience is an appealing solution for working nurses. With a laptop computer or mobile device and connection to the Internet, students can do class work anywhere and anytime.

Other advantages of online courses include the following:

- Multiple media formats resulting in greater matching of instruction to learning styles
- Active student involvement
- Individualized and collaborative learning
- Information linked to student pace and performance
- Just-in-time instructional assistance
- On-time assessment, feedback, and reinforcement
- Optimal use of instructor's expertise
- Access to online libraries, databases, and learning resources
- Ability to network with colleagues in specialty areas without geographic limitations

Distance education will not meet the needs of all nurses; however, it is ideal for the individual who is motivated, needs flexibility, and wants to maintain professional accountability through self-evaluation and ongoing education. Online education is a learning option based on the assumption that students will become a part of a community of learners even as they work separately from each other and their instructors.

Limitations of Online Education

Online courses do have some limitations; eight key issues are presented here. First, students must have access to a computer or mobile device and an Internet service. Although cellular telephone service with smartphones has lessened the technology gap, there are still many individuals who lack such access. If students must drive to use on-campus computer labs, several of the key advantages of online courses are lost. Second, some students are still not computer literate; for them this modality may be ineffective. However, this limitation is rapidly declining as more people worldwide become computer and Internet literate. During the next 10 years, virtually all undergraduate college students will have grown up using computers and the Internet in school. Most prospective graduate students will come to school already using the Internet in their personal lives or in their jobs. They will feel as comfortable with Internet communications as they do with face-to-face communication.

Third, although the Internet is quite adaptable to most theory courses, there remain many challenges to teaching hands-on skills content through this medium. The use of simulations can be an important technology to reduce this problem. However, little replaces hands-on learning experiences when technical skills need to be developed. Even though the problem of teaching hands-on skills in online courses has not been resolved, there is also a need for teachers to personally coach students to enhance clinical reasoning in the practice of nursing. Coaching can be accomplished using distance education technologies, but clinical reasoning must be carefully nurtured with an authentic presence of the teacher in the learning process.

Fourth, some teachers are not yet sufficiently familiar with the online format as an educational tool to function well. Some are highly resistant to online teaching, and some are not well suited to teaching online. Just as students should assess themselves for readiness to learn online, faculty should assess themselves for their readiness to teach online.

Fifth, some teachers continue to be extremely concerned about the possible loss of learning of certain types of content due to the loss of face-to-face class discussions. The evidence, to date, shows that online learning equals and sometimes exceeds learning in the traditional classroom format (Shachar & Neumann, 2010). The many concerns about lower learning for students in online courses have not been validated—learning levels in both modalities are highly dependent upon student commitment to learning.

Sixth, the teacher needs to be intimately involved with assisting first-time students in getting started successfully and to work to keep students from dropping out of classes. This is especially true of continuing education courses but is also true with degree-seeking students. Only the teacher knows if the student is active in the course, so only the teacher can perform this student-retention activity. Although it is understandable that faculty might believe that adult learners can take care of themselves, problems that seem overwhelming to students might be resolved easily by the teacher. Distance education courses and programs depend on fully engaged instructors in order to have successful outcomes.

Seventh, authentication of student work can be problematic in online courses. Teachers always have to be concerned that grades are based on work completed by students enrolled in the class without assistance of others. Unfortunately, online courses do not offer any better protections against dishonesty than do classroom courses (Hart & Morgan, 2010). Sewell, Frith, and Colvin (2010) provide reasonable approaches to academic honesty, examination security, and plagiarism prevention in their discussion of summative evaluation. Faculty in a department or college should agree on a minimum set of principles to enhance academic honesty of students.

Finally, online classes require infrastructure and human resources to support students and teachers. In order to have good distance-education programs, postsecondary institutions have to invest in high-bandwidth networks, purchase LMSs, provide technical support for students and teachers, provide professional development for faculty, hire instructional designers to work with faculty who teach classes, and manage enrollment in online courses in a manner that supports frequent student–faculty communication. The investment by colleges and universities is not only up-front; it is also continuous. For example, students are most likely to have difficulty the first week of class, and that is when extra support staff members need to be available by phone and e-mail. Because students are just as likely to be online at 1 a.m. as they are at 9 a.m., around-the-clock support services are critical.

IMPORTANT THEMES

There are several themes that shape online education and the future direction of learning and teaching. These themes, initially developed by Kearsley (2000), are all interrelated and overlapping but important for the potential student.

1. *Collaboration:* The single biggest change that the Internet brings to education is the increased collaboration between students and teachers, which includes diverse individuals in all parts of the world. Many activities and projects in online classes involve information seeking and sharing. Even when there is no specific intent to collaborate, it often happens anyway because it is so easy to interact online.
2. *Connectivity:* Though closely related to collaboration, connectivity relates to the way that individuals interact with each other using discussion forums, chat rooms, instant messaging, text, e-mail, Tweeting, Facebook, and many other ways. Whether using a smartphone, tablet, laptop computer, desktop computer, television, or other mobile device, when the Internet is just a click away, teachers and students can easily connect across time and geographic locations. Connectivity also includes the way that individuals connect with information. Rapid access to research reports, systematic reviews of research, and clinical guidelines helps embed evidence-based practice in the delivery of patient care.
3. *Student-centeredness:* When experienced nurses return to school for further formal education, they respond well to a program that is based on adult learning principles. These principles, developed by Malcolm Knowles (1980), are based on the assumption that the student is a capable decision maker and is an active participant rather than a passive receiver in the teaching–learning process. Teachers must recognize the value of a less hierarchical learning environment and embrace the role of facilitator as their primary function. One of the most important contributions of this work is to increase awareness of the learner's rightful place at the center of the instructional process.
4. *Unboundedness:* The Internet offers online education that eliminates the walls of the classroom. It gives students access to information and people anywhere in the world. Online education removes boundaries having to do with where and when students learn as well as who can be a learner. This is especially important for continuing education for professional nurses.
5. *Virtual community:* A sense of community is important, whether it is the community of learners defined by a particular school or continuing education program or a professional nursing organization. The Internet makes it possible to define virtual communities around common interests and work-related activities.

A community is possible only if a sense of presence is created. Audio and sound are important in creating presence.

6. *Exploration:* The Internet allows learners to integrate knowledge into their own behavior and belief system and to create new knowledge and insight that can come only when there is the adventure of discovery. Many online activities involve adventure or discovery learning. Problem-based learning is an example of this type of learning activity.
7. *Shared knowledge:* Nursing professionals and students can tap into a vast knowledge network, and they can contribute as well. Information on the Internet is immediately available to anyone in the world at any time. Sharing knowledge is the core of education, but prior to computer networks, this was accomplished only in limited ways.
8. *Multisensory experience:* Learning theories tell us that learning is more effective when it involves multiple sensory channels such as visuals, color, movement, sound, voice, touch, and smell. For example, Edgar Dale's classic cone-of-experience theory suggests that individuals learn approximately 10% of read material, 50% of observed demonstrations and material read, and 80% of material that is interactive (Dale, 1969). Multimedia technology is available on the Internet and can provide most kinds of learning experiences except for touch and smell. Although these experiences may not be perfect, they are often much better than traditional learning activities that are primarily based on lectures.
9. *Authenticity:* Internet education is highly authentic in nature. Students can work with nurse experts as they explore solutions to real problems. This gives the educational experience relevance to the learning needs of the student. The Internet provides direct access to major repositories of research studies, systematic reviews of research, clinical guidelines, and actual databases holding rich health care information.

WHAT TO EXPECT WITH ONLINE LEARNING

Until recently, the primary function of a teacher has been to transfer knowledge, with the student in a passive role. Most teaching and learning is passive, and most students find this style of learning very safe and comfortable. Distance education students and teachers need to be prepared for a change in this approach. When the Internet becomes the primary vehicle for learners to receive information and skills, classes that primarily transfer information become obsolete. Instead, the student becomes an active participant in the process. The role of the instructor is to make the information meaningful, create a positive learning environment, integrate knowledge into the learner's own belief system, and create new knowledge and insight that come when learners are engaged in intense discussion and exploration. In so doing, a community of learners is "present" in the virtual classroom.

In some programs, clinical skills are evaluated by connecting students to instructors, using portable videoconferencing devices such as webcam technology with two-way videoconferencing. Those teaching in online learning environments must be prepared to deliver instruction with various online learning modalities in order to meet the diverse learning styles of individuals, similar to the preparations that are adopted in the traditional classroom setting for students with various learning styles. Technology and its applications in education change quickly; even experienced online teachers have learning curves.

SUMMARY AND KEY POINTS

The academic quality and legitimacy of well-designed and well-executed distance education programs have been shown to match or exceed traditional classroom settings. Furthermore, the recent acceleration of enrollments in distance education has widespread implications for nursing faculty and the students they teach. Both must embrace different teacher–student roles. As students become more responsible for their knowledge development, they gain key skills to stay abreast of rapidly changing advances in nursing science and in the delivery of health care.

- Distance education is planned learning where teachers and students are physically and sometimes temporally separated
- Online education has moved to the forefront of distance education
- Web-enhanced, hybrid, and completely online courses use the Internet to deliver instruction
- Asynchronous learning occurs when students access and interact in a course at different times, whereas in synchronous learning, they access and interact in real time
- Nurse educators can achieve transformative education in online classes. They can enhance collaboration, provide connectivity, be

student-centered, provide education unbounded by place and time, create virtual communities, support exploration and inquiry, promote sharing of knowledge, create multisensory experiences, and create highly authentic education

REFERENCES

Allen, E., & Seaman, J. (2011). *Going the distance: Online education in the United States, 2011*. Babson Park, MA: Babson Survey Research Group. Retrieved from http://www.onlinelearningsurvey.com/reports/goingthedistance.pdf.

Benner, P., Sutphen, M., Leonard, V., & Day, L. (2010). *Educating nurses: A call for radical transformation*. San Francisco, CA: John Wiley and Sons.

Briggs, L. (2010). Immersive distance learning to boost retention. *Campus Technology*. Retrieved from http://campustechnology.com/Articles/2010/06/09/Immersive-Distance-Learning-To-Boost-Retention.aspx?Page=1

Commission on Collegiate Nursing Education (CCNE). (2009). *Standards for accreditation of baccalaureate and graduate degree nursing programs* (Amended April 2009). Retrieved from http://www.aacn.nche.edu/ccne-accreditation/standards09.pdf

Dale, E. (1969). *Audiovisual methods in teaching* (3rd ed.). New York, NY: Holt, Rinehart & Winston.

Escoffery, C., Miner, K. R., & Alperin, M. (2003). Ten informative web sites on distance education. *American Journal of Health Behavior, 27*, 464–465.

Hart, L., & Morgan, L. (2010). Academic integrity in an online registered nurse to baccalaureate in nursing program. *Journal of Continuing Education in Nursing, 41*(11), 498–505. doi:10.3928/00220124-20100701-03

Holden, J. & Westfall, P. (2010). *An Instructional Media Selection Guide for Distance Learning* – Implications for Blended Learning Featuring an Introduction to Virtual Worlds. Boston, MA: United States Distance Learning Association.

Institute of Medicine. (2011). *The future of nursing: Leading change, advancing health*. Washington, DC: The National Academies Press. Retrieved from https://download.nap.edu/catalog.php?record_id=12956

Instructional Technology Council (ITC). (2011). *2010 distance education survey results. Trends in eLearning: Tracking the impact of eLearning at community colleges*. Washington, DC: Instructional Technology Council. Retrieved from http://www.itcnetwork.org/attachments/article/87/ITCAnnualSurveyMay2011Final.pdf

Johnson, L., Smith, R., Willis, H., Levine, A., & Haywood, K., (2011). *The 2011 horizon report*. Austin, TX: The New Media Consortium. Retrieved from http://wp.nmc.org/horizon2011/

Kearsley, G. (2000). *Online education: Learning and teaching in cyberspace*. Belmont, CA: Wadsworth/Thomson Learning.

Knowles, M. S. (1980). *The modern practice of adult education: From pedagogy to androgogy*. Chicago, IL: Follett.

Marcyjanik, D., & Zom, C. R. (2011). Accessibility in online nursing education for persons with disability. *Nurse Educator, 36*(6), 241–245. doi:10.1097/NNE.0b013e3182333f9d

National Center for Education Statistics (NCES). (2011). *The condition of education 2011* (NCES 2011-033, Indicator 43). Retrieved from http://nces.ed.gov/programs/coe/index.asp

National Council of State Boards of Nursing. (n.d.). *Distance learning/web definitions: A resource for the model education rules*. Retrieved from https://www.ncsbn.org/836.htm

National League for Nursing Accreditation Commission. (2008). *Accreditation manual.* Retrieved from http://www.nlnac.org/manuals/NLNACManual2008.pdf

Parsad, L., & Lewis, L. (2008). *Distance education at degree-granting postsecondary institutions: 2006–07. First look December 2008* (NCES 2009–044). U.S. Department of Education. National Center for Education Statistics. Washington, DC. Retrieved from http://nces.ed.gov/pubs2009/2009044.pdf

Paulus, T., Myers, C., Mixer, S., Wyatt, T., Lee, D., & Lee, J. (2010). For faculty, by faculty: A case study of learning to teach online. *International Journal of Nursing Education Scholarship*, *7*(1). doi:10.2202/1548-923X.1979

Raths, D. (2012). IT trends to watch in 2012. *Campus Technology*. Retrieved from http://campustechnology.com/Articles/2012/01/01/Whats-Hot-Whats-Not-Extra.aspx?Page=1

Sewell, J., Frith, K. H., & Colvin, M. (2010). Online assessment strategies: A primer. *Journal of Online Learning and Teaching, 6*(1), 1–10. Retrieved from http://jolt.merlot.org/vol6no1/sewell_0310.pdf

Shachar, M., & Neumann, Y. (2010) Twenty years of research on the academic performance differences between traditional and distance learning. *MERLOT Journal of Online Learning and Teaching, 6*(2). Retrieved from http://jolt.merlot.org/vol6no2/shachar_0610.pdf

Sheehy, K. (2012, January 10). U.S. news ranks top online degree programs. *U.S. News & World Report*. Retrieved from http://www.usnews.com/education/online-education/articles/2012/01/10/us-news-ranks-top-online-degree-programs

Simonson, M. (2008). *Distance Learning: Key Terms You Might Want to Know.* North Miami Beach, FL: Nova Southeastern University, Fischler School of Education. Retrieved from http://www.usdla.org/assets/pdf_files/Glossary_Distance.pdf.

THREE

Faculty Preparation for Teaching Online

ARLENE E. JOHNSON and NANCY K. MEEHAN

The introduction of online learning into nursing education has transformed the role of the nurse educator. This chapter will address many of the issues that are of concern to nursing faculty who teach online, including readiness to teach, competencies, self-assessment, preparation, course design strategies, essentials of a successful online course, the advantages and challenges of teaching online, and practical hints.

There are a number of issues that faculty face when moving to online teaching. Transitioning from a face-to-face course to an online course may be seen as a threatening experience (Grant & Thornton, 2007). Faculty are concerned about the technology skill set necessary to successfully create and manage an online course. Time to migrate a course online is limited. Many faculty without formal training are not aware of or have misunderstood the tools available to create an online course and simply adapt their face-to-face course for the online environment with limited success (Bates & Poole, 2003). Faculty need training and assistance to transition from teaching in the traditional face-to-face classroom to teaching in an online environment (Taylor & McQuiggan, 2008; Ko & Rossen, 2010). Yet, faculty preparation for teaching online varies considerably. Palloff and Pratt (2011) proposed a systems approach to faculty development for online teaching, the Best System for Online Faculty Development Model, reflecting interaction between faculty development, self-development, and institutional support.

FACULTY READINESS FOR TEACHING ONLINE

Teaching and Learning: A Shift in Pedagogy

One of the most significant issues that emerged in the shift from traditional classroom instruction to teaching online is the faculty's readiness to teach. Lack of technology knowledge is often identified as a barrier, but the shift in pedagogy often becomes even more significant as faculty move to the online teaching environment. Instructors who feel confident in the face-to-face classroom may experience feelings of inadequacy or nervousness when teaching online.

Experienced online faculty reported that in order to teach in the web-based environment, they rethought their philosophies of teaching and learning (Robina & Anderson, 2010; Johnson, 2008). Macy (2007) described a nursing faculty's transition from face-to-face teaching as going from an "A teacher" in the classroom to a "C teacher" online. Robina and Anderson (2010) examined the variables the affect nursing faculty efficacy levels and participation in online teaching and found that years of general teaching experience did not correlate with a nursing faculty member's online teaching efficacy. Robina and Anderson found that instructors who reported the highest levels of online teaching efficacy had taught at least three online courses, received satisfactory preparation, and had instructional designer support and/or colleague support. Novice online instructors identified faculty and experience in taking an online course as important. Only a small number (18%) of faculty who participated in the study had received release time.

There is a dynamic relationship among content, pedagogy, and technology (Koehler, Mishra, Hershey, & Peruski, 2004). An effective online teaching pedagogy uses learning theories in course design, including constructivism and adult learning. The nurse educator role is transformed from knowledge deliverer to facilitator, and students engage in collaborative learning experiences to develop new knowledge. The nurse educator who teaches in distance education guides students through a transformative learning experience as adult learners using a teaching strategy called *scaffolding*, which is consistent with constructivism (Collison, Elbaum, Haavind, & Tinker, 2000; Holly, Legg, Mueller, & Adelman, 2008; Legg, Aldeman, & Levitt, 2009). Adults are more likely to actively participate in learning situations that are meaningful to them and prefer an active versus passive learning environment (Palloff & Pratt, 2011). The online classroom diffuses authority and places the student at the center of the learning process (Alexander, Polyakova-Norwood, Johnston, Christensen, & Loquist, 2003). To achieve this, the instructor must relinquish a certain amount of control. When the instructor assumes a facilitator/participant role, students are guided toward a deeper level of investigation and inquiry (Collison et al., 2000).

Savery and Duffy (2006) suggested the following principles to develop a constructivist approach to teaching online:

1. Anchoring all learning activities to a larger task or problem
2. Supporting learners in developing ownership of the overall problem or task
3. Designing an authentic task and learning environment to reflect the complexity of the environment in which learners should be able to function at the end of learning
4. Giving learners ownership of the process used to develop a solution
5. Designing the learning environment to support and challenge the learners' thinking
6. Encouraging the testing of ideas against alternative views and alternative contexts
7. Providing an opportunity for and support of reflection on both content and learning process

A well-designed online classroom provides a social experience; as such, the degree of social presence is an important pedagogical consideration (Holly et al., 2008; Mayne & Wu, 2011). Faculty–student relationships in the online classroom are different from those in the face-to-face classroom. Some instructors report that they have experienced stronger relationships with students in the online environment, while others report feeling more distant (Johnson, 2008; Ryan, Carlton, & Ali, 2004). Confident students in a traditional classroom may find themselves intimidated in the online environment. The introverted student may actually flourish in the online classroom. A lack of social cues can lead to misunderstandings or behaviors that might not occur when people are in a face-to-face environment. Mayne and Wu (2011) suggested several strategies for establishing social presence including personal e-mail contact by the instructor prior to beginning the course, clearly defined evaluation methods, identified roles of the instructor and students, and frequent communication between teacher and students.

Competencies for Teaching Online

Covington, Petherbridge, and Warren (2005) described a triangulated model of support for faculty making the transition to online teaching, including administrative support, peer support, and professional development. Administrative support would include designated funds for equipment needed to teach online, including hardware, software, and technology support during hours students would be accessing their online courses. In the ideal situation, administrators provide release from some other responsibilities while faculty is designing a new online course. The power of peers to support novice online teachers is particularly powerful when there is a shared experience of learning new technology skills or discussing online teaching pedagogy in professional development activities.

When faced with an assignment to teach an online course, many are concerned about their level of technological expertise. The ideal team to convert a traditional face-to-face class to an online class would include the course instructor and an instructional technology support person. The technology competencies necessary to teach online are the abilities to (a) set up folders and directories; (b) use word processing software (cut, copy, paste, save files); (c) handle e-mail communications, including attachments; and (d) use a browser to access the World Wide Web (Ko & Rossen, 2010). Once basic competencies are met, nurse educators can become more creative by adding social media, video and audio, and simulations.

Online courses are most often taught using an online course delivery platform (also known as learning management system [LMS] or course management system [CMS]), such as WebCT©, Blackboard©, or Educator©, that can be accessed via the Internet. Many of the platforms have built-in web authoring tools that allow the faculty to create web pages without the need to know HTML (hypertext markup language). These tools are "pedagogically advanced platforms," which provide a variety of synchronous and asynchronous tools that can be used in online courses (Moore, Winograd, & Lange, 2001). Included in many of the platforms are mechanisms for online testing and assessment, as well as the capability to track the progress of students. For example, Blackboard Learn© allows tracking of data that enable the instructor to view when and how often each student accesses content pages.

Faculty Self-Assessment

Many assessment tools exist for faculty to evaluate their readiness to teach online. Some tools focus on whether a teacher has the technical skills necessary to teach online (Online Teaching Resources, 2011). Other assessment tools try to gauge a teacher's readiness for teaching online by combining technical knowledge with organization skills (Paradise Community College, n.d.). Still other assessment tools evaluate whether the faculty's teaching style is suited to online teaching (Teaching Styles Quiz, 2001). Assessment of Faculty Readiness to Teach Online includes the ability of faculty members to adjust their teaching style to the online environment (Palloff & Pratt, 2011). Another self-assessment tool, Faculty Self-Assessment for Online Teaching, evaluates faculty preparedness in four categories: (a) organization and time management, (b) communicating online, (c) teaching and online experience, and (d) technical skills (Pennsylvania State University, 2009). The Pennsylvania State assessment is taken online and gives feedback that could be invaluable in the quest to become an excellent online teacher. The result is a score for each criterion (e.g., detail oriented) as well as feedback that can includes resources for further reading.

One of the first things that a nurse educator must acknowledge is the time necessary to teach online and organizational skills. In a study by Keeton (2004), faculty "agreed that teaching well online is more time-consuming than teaching face-to-face" (p. 77). Cavanaugh (2006) compared the same course taught online versus face to face. Results showed that preparation for the online course took 35 hours, while that for the face-to-face course took 3 hours; teaching the online course took 73 hours, while the face-to-face course took 27 hours; and online office hours took 44 hours compared to 32 face-to-face hours. Worley and Tesdell (2009) categorized teaching-related activities as prep time and effort, teaching time and effort, technical time and effort, as well as others. In this study, setting up an online environment, record keeping, and other miscellaneous activities took significantly more time in the online courses than the face-to-face course. The biggest time commitment for an online course is the up-front course development. Even the smallest details should be recognized before the course begins. The second biggest time commitment is ongoing communication with each student followed by consistent check-in for online discussion, and so on. Good organizational skills keep the course running smoothly. Requisite skills include grading assignments using rubrics, responding to student e-mails within an agreed-upon timeframe, and keeping electronic records in an electronic filing system for easy access.

A second category that is addressed in both self-assessments is experiences with online teaching. Most faculty members report the benefit of having taken an online class themselves. By reviewing other faculty members' online courses or inviting an expert in distance education to review a course before going "live," some problems can be avoided. Also, it is important to pursue the textbook publisher's resources and resources available on the Internet for online teaching; it is imperative that content permission be addressed. Teachers must obtain the appropriate copyright permissions for all the materials used in the online course.

A third area assessed by both tools is technical skills. Technical skills can include e-mail skills, computer proficiency, Internet proficiency, software skills, typing skills, course management proficiency, and patience with technology. More advanced online technical skills may include blogging, writing a wiki, and using social networking sites that also contribute to knowledge because these can be done outside the class on the Internet.

Being an effective online communicator includes activities such as providing clear written instructions to students for assignments and expected outcomes, conveying personality, and using an engaging tone in written language. The Pennsylvania State collaborators feel that communicating in writing is one of the most important skills for teaching online. Finding a motivational and engaging tone of voice in writing can be challenging, but it is a rewarding skill to build in the online classroom. The University of Michigan's Project IDEAL consortium website provides some valid advice on communicating in the online classroom in the video "Voice of Experience" (www.projectideal.org/getting_started/teaching.html). The use of humor in the online classroom is a delicate issue because of the lack of body language and sound of the human voice to know that the statement was supposed to be humorous. Written messages in the online classroom or via e-mail are scrutinized by the reader and may be misinterpreted.

An additional category is attitudes toward online learning. Taylor (2003) believes that "some of the most critical barriers to change in educational processes are personal ones" (p. 76). In fact, faculty beliefs and expectations about teaching can hinder their ability to change their teaching practices (Sunal et al., 2001). Trusting that lecture is not the only way to convey course content and that student-centered activities (reading, discussion, and assignments) can result in student learning and accomplishment of the course objectives is critical to success in the online classroom. The online teacher must be certain that learning is occurring and is measured by credible means.

One area not discussed in either the Palloff and Pratt (2011) tool or the Pennsylvania State tool is teaching style (Teaching Styles Quiz, 2001). Teaching style categories include formal authority, demonstrator or personal model, delegator, and facilitator. Teachers with a formal authority teaching style use primarily teacher-centered strategies. This is usually the "sage on the stage" model. The demonstrator or personal model style tends to be teacher-centered but has an emphasis on demonstration. The delegator style is one wherein a teacher acts as a consultant, giving students a choice of projects. The final style, facilitator, focuses on learning activities and is a student-centered style that encourages independent learning. Developing the skills to facilitate learning is the goal of becoming an online educator.

Types of Preparation

The majority of faculty at higher education institutions educate themselves about online teaching instead of undergoing formal training. In 2001, 63% of business faculty indicated they learned to develop online courses on their own, while in 2006, 74% claimed they were self-taught (Perreault, Waldman, Alexander, & Zhao, 2008). In a study to learn more about the needs of faculty who will teach online courses, Taylor and McQuiggan (2008) found that, when designing and developing online courses, faculty were most interested in topics such as choosing appropriate technology, converting course material, creating effective online assessment instruments, creating video clips, and assessing student progress. Topics of concern to faculty that focused specifically on course delivery were facilitating discussion forums, building and enhancing faculty–student relationships in the online environment, facilitating web conferencing sessions, increasing interactions, managing online teaching workloads, and providing meaningful feedback on assignments.

Faculty learning needs are as variable as student learning needs; therefore, a combination of professional development activities could be the best approach. The content for faculty development should include both technical training and pedagogical training. Technical training should include the CMS that the institution uses as well as other software that can assist with online communication. Pedagogical training can include best practices of online education, facilitating interaction, discussion, active learning, and collaboration online; evaluating online courses; as well as building communities (Pankowski, 2004). Another component of faculty development is content. Koehler et al. (2004) describe content as the actual subject matter.

Covington et al. (2005) describe a comprehensive triangulated support approach that includes administrative support, professional development support, and peer support for faculty. This collaborative approach removes several obstacles that include resolving administrative issues and ensuring appropriate resources and peer support as well as support for adequate professional development. Pankowski (2004) included the additional components of mentoring and online course work.

Some institutions require mandatory training for all faculty who teach an online course. These programs vary. Montgomery College has an intensive 6-week online program built on the principles of Quality Matters (M. Mills, personal communication, August 30, 2011). Dallas Baptist University has a 6-month face-to-face course where faculty meet with a course developer to create their first online course. Before first-time instructors teach online, they take a 2-hour online pedagogy training course (K. Shelton, personal communication, August 30, 2011). Some programs are voluntary, such as a 10-week "eLearning in Higher Education" module at the University of Birmingham (2012). Indiana University (2011) provides streaming video and synchronized slides. Purdue University provides a distance education mentoring program (DEMP; Barczyk, Buckenmeyer, & Feldman, 2010; Hixon & Zamojski, 2010).

ONLINE COURSE DESIGN STRATEGIES

After self-assessment for learning needs and teaching style, review of pedagogy for online learning, and improvement of technology skills, particularly those that promote communication in online courses, nurse educators can focus on designing the course. The first strategy is to seek out templates for online courses at the institution. Often, these templates include such elements as syllabi, course organization, layout of course pages, and guidelines for font type and size. Templates can prove invaluable. If the institution does not have templates, samples are available on the Internet.

Faculty members must consider the diversity of students who might access their courses. Using the principles of universal design, online courses should be planned with both usability and accessibility in mind. Universal design is "an approach to the design of all products and environments to be as usable as possible by as many people as possible regardless of age, ability, or situation" (Universal Design Education, n.d., para. 1). The University of Connecticut's Universal Design for Instruction (UDI) Online provides a chart of many easy-to-use e-tools, their features, their limitations, and ideas for use with online courses and universal design ("UDI Online," 2011).

In order to design the best online course using universal design strategies, the University of Arkansas at Little Rock (n.d.) gives 10 simple steps. They are:

1. *Content first, then design:* Determine what content should be included, and use outlines or concept maps for good flow of content.
2. *Provide simple, consistent navigation:* Be consistent throughout the entire course and use concise, meaningful text for links. Provide a table of contents for easy navigation to all parts of the course. Use consistent design, order, and naming for files as well as content folders throughout the course. Make due dates obvious. The course home page should be professional, attractive, interesting, as well as easy to understand.
3. *Include an accommodation statement:* Place an accommodation statement in your syllabus or primary course page and make sure a link to your disability services website.
4. *Know your CMS tools:* Many CMS tools create challenges for students as they learn to use the system to accomplish their learning. Advanced features such as online testing, chat, and student presentation software can be difficult for students due to technical problems or student unease. Real-time chat sessions can create barriers for students with learning disabilities.
5. *Model and teach good discussion-board etiquette:* Provide students with netiquette tips as well as discussion-board guidelines to help the students have a professional presence in the course.
6. *Use color with care:* Provide good color contrast and do not use color to convey meaning. Students who are color-blind or prefer to work from printed material using a black-and-white printer will not be aware of the color of the text (Kyrnin, 2012).
7. *Provide accessible document formats:* Web pages designed in HTML are an ideal format for providing information online. When the formatting of a page is important, the instructor can use portable document format (PDF); however, the file size should be appropriate for downloading across a variety of Internet connection speeds.
8. *Choose fonts carefully:* Online learners have an immense amount of reading, including online course materials, e-books, e-mail, and Internet searches. Clean and simple fonts such as Arial or Helvetica are good choices. Limit bold and italics, and avoid all-capital letters.
9. *Think differently about multimedia:* A variety of forms of multimedia can include text, images, audio, and video. Multimedia can increase the level of student engagement because it appeals to various learning styles. Multimedia is best used for parts of the course that remain the same over time.

10. *Employ rubrics and usability testing to evaluate course design:* Rubrics can make good course assessment tools for the design of an online course (Lunney & Sammarco, 2009; California State University, Chico, 2009).

Once the basics of universal design have been taken into consideration, the next focus should be overall online course design. Hudson Valley Community College (n.d.) provides some best practices of online course design that include additional online course design strategies not mentioned earlier. These include the following:

1. *Syllabus*: The online course syllabus is similar to an on-site syllabus. The instructor's contact information should include an e-mail address and Skype contact name in addition to cell phone and office phone numbers. The course calendar should be included or added as a separate document in the course. The lateness policy should be clear and may be different from that in a face-to-face course. Since the syllabus will be in HTML, providing hyperlinks in the syllabus to resources that are important to student success should be used. Good links to provide may be the course website, instructor website, online library, and technical support personnel.
2. *Course materials*: Today, electronic textbooks (e-books) are commonly used in online classes. Clear instructions are needed for downloading/saving the textbook and finding the associated publisher materials that support the textbook.
3. *Teacher presence*: Presence in online courses can be created using e-mail and a conversational tone in course materials and in posts to students. Some teachers use an avatar to add interest and a personal touch to the class. All of these strategies have a positive effect on student satisfaction (Shea, Fredericksen, Pickett, & Pelz, 2003).
4. *Orientation of students*: The first online course that students take requires more instructions and patience from the teacher. Orientation can include a range of activities to provide practice in using tools in the learning management system.
5. *Feedback*: Students should know when their assignments will be graded (typically within 5 days of submission) and how to find their grades and feedback.
6. *Discussions*: If the course includes discussion questions, a review of instructions and grading criteria is helpful. A grading rubric is a preferred method to use for discussion questions. A grading rubric provides information about length, quality, references, and scholarly rigor for the discussion question responses.

7. *Assessments*: Ways for students to assess their knowledge and skills and provide feedback to the instructor should be built into online courses. Consider self-assessment tests, quizzes, and an end-of-course survey assessing student perception of their course achievements. Sewell, Frith, and Colvin (2010) provide a primer for online assessment strategies that tie directly to the course outcomes and teaching methods.

Another area of concern when looking at online course design is the instructional activities that are best suited for the online environment. Ko and Rossen (2010) discuss several student activities that are appropriate for an online course. Some frequently used instructional activities are group activities, role-playing and simulations, summaries and/or consensus groups, evidence-based lab assignments, reflective activities, online discussions, scenarios and case studies, peer editing, guest speakers, cross-cultural experiences, and a variety of interactive websites.

WHAT MAKES AN ONLINE COURSE SUCCESSFUL?

Community Building

To maximize the learning experience in the online classroom, specific attention must be given to developing a sense of community. The learning community becomes the vehicle through which learning occurs (Palloff & Pratt, 2011). A strong sense of community in the online classroom leads to enhancement of student engagement and ultimately improved learning outcomes (Gallagher-Lepak, Reilly, & Killion, 2009). A dynamic community model supports an environment that promotes inquiry and supports learning (Keeton, 2004). Helping students to become comfortable with expressing their thoughts and feelings in writing is key to a successful online environment. To create a social presence in the online classroom, the instructor can model inclusion of feelings in written communications. When an instructor is successful in fostering community, students report they have a better learning experience, feel closer to their peers, and get to know their instructors better than they ever did in a traditional classroom (Lynch, 2002).

Faculty should incorporate learning strategies that result in meaningful interactions between students and instructors. Thurmond and Wambach (2004) discussed three types of interaction in the online classroom: learner–instructor interaction, learner–content interaction, and learner–learner interaction. Learner–instructor interaction is highly desired by learners. During learner–instructor interaction, the instructor should seek to stimulate the learner's interest in the course content as well as encourage self-direction and self-motivation. Learner–content interaction is the process of the learner intellectually interacting with content that results in changes in the cognitive structures of the learner's mind. Learner–learner interaction occurs with or without the presence of the instructor and can take place between two learners or among a group of learners. Collaborative learning activities allow learners to achieve a deeper level of knowledge generation. The most powerful experiences may be those in which interaction occurs with all group members instead of between one participant and a facilitator in a group setting. Through learner-to-learner interaction and collaborative learning experiences, students develop a sense of community as they discover socially constructed meaning (Palloff & Pratt, 2003, 2011).

When asked what makes an online educator exceptional, nursing students described exemplary online educators as challengers, affirmers, and persons of influence. Students appreciated educators who had high expectations for themselves and those who challenged students to perform at high levels. Affirmation and encouragement to students during the course was also important. Finally, the students valued instructors who were experts in their subject area and those who gave constructive, relative feedback (Edwards, Perry, & Janzen, 2011).

Collaboration

The Institute of Medicine (2003) defined core competencies for nursing education, including the ability to work in interdisciplinary teams. Teamwork and collaboration are essential skills that nursing students must develop to effectively engage in quality interdisciplinary care (Long, 2003). Collaborative teamwork including open communication, mutual respect, and shared decision making will result in quality patient care (Cronenwett et al., 2007). The online classroom is an optimal environment for development of collaboration skills in nursing education. Chickering and Ehrmann (1996) proposed that teamwork in the classroom develops reciprocity and cooperation among students. When students work collaboratively, deeper levels of understanding and critical evaluation of the subject matter may develop. Spontaneous collaboration may emerge as students begin to feel they are part of a supportive learning community (Palloff & Pratt, 2003).

Collaboration has been identified as an important component of online education, but collaborative learning is often not reflected in online courses. Most online courses require students to participate in online discussion, which gives an equal voice to all participants, and asynchronous discussion, which allows students to reflect on classmates' comments while creating their own contribution to the discussion (Harasim, 1990; Levin, Kim, & Riel, 1990; Zsohar & Smith, 2008). When using collaborative learning in an online class, the faculty member carefully defines the learning goals of the collaboration activity and how students' participation will be assessed (Swan, Shen, & Hiltz, 2006; Zsohar & Smith, 2008). An effective collaborative activity requires that the students not only actively engage in the activity but also reflect on the learning process. Faculty must set the stage for collaboration, create assignments that allow students to work from their areas of strength, model collaboration, and effectively evaluate the process.

Connectivity

Participating in an online class, whether as a faculty member or as a student, allows 24/7 connection to the class and the other members of the learning community. Technology, particularly use of mobile devices, is a common method of connectivity with many students staying socially connected (Mastrian, McGonigle, Mahan, & Bixler, 2011). Although students can be "net savvy," they still need guidance about the quality and reliability of Internet resources (Skiba & Barton, 2006).

PRACTICAL HINTS FOR TEACHING ONLINE

There are a number of educators who have published best-practice recommendations for teaching online. Chickering and Gamson (1987) identified "Seven Principles for Good Practice in Undergraduate Education" that were later applied to teaching with technology by Chickering and Ehrmann (1996) in "Implementing the Seven Principles: Technology as Lever":

1. Good practice encourages contact between students and faculty. The use of technology in the classroom can actually strengthen faculty–student interactions. Asynchronous communication allows the student and faculty member to thoughtfully compose their

communication and may provide the student with an increased sense of intimacy and be less intimidating than live communication in the classroom. The asynchronous environment may result in a higher caliber of classroom discussion.

2. Good practice develops reciprocity and cooperation among students. Computer-based learning provides students with increased opportunities to communicate through online discussions that require responses to peers and group projects.
3. Good practice uses active learning technologies. A variety of simulation experiences are available for implementation into courses.
4. Good practice gives prompt feedback. When students are learning in a distance environment, it is important for the instructor to be actively engaged with the class as a whole and to provide prompt, constructive feedback to students on their performance.
5. Good practice emphasizes time on task. If used efficiently, technology can significantly improve time on task for both faculty members and students.
6. Good practice communicates high expectations. It is important to clearly identify expectations for course work and class participation. Student assignments can be subjected to peer evaluation, which may ultimately lead to increased performance.
7. Good practice respects diverse talents and ways of learning. Distance technologies offer students an additional platform for demonstrating mastery of competencies and an opportunity to take more responsibility for their learning.

Authenticity and Academic Integrity

One of the identified student issues associated with online education is academic integrity (Bristol, 2005; Fehn, 2005; Hurt, 2008; Johnson, 2005). Cheating on online exams and assignments is a major concern (Hurt, 2008; Rowe, 2004). Instructors must create safeguards to ensure that students are held to the same standards of academic integrity as students who learn in traditional classrooms. The means to measure student mastery of course outcomes may have to be modified in the online environment. Learning outcomes and strategies should be linked to methods that will be used to assess students' mastery of competencies (Palloff & Pratt, 2003).

The two most common issues of academic honesty in online learning are identity crisis and plagiarism. Identity crisis refers to the issue of how the teacher knows the person online is the person who registered for the class. The identity problem is difficult to address because the complex technology needed to identify an individual in a remote setting is very expensive. It would be prudent to create original and unique course activities and assessments that make it more difficult for students to cheat. When plagiarism is suspected, it is suggested that the faculty confirm with factual evidence. There are numerous tools for detecting plagiarism in online courses, including Turnitin© (turnitin.com) and wCopyfind© (plagiarism.bloomfieldmedia.com/z-wordpress/software/wcopyfind). An academic honesty policy should be included in the course syllabus.

Acxiom (2009) provides an overview of ways to verify student identity using electronic methods such as passwords, biometrics and/or web recordings, a web videoconference proctor, and face-to-face proctored exams. The Higher Education Opportunity Act (United States Department of Education, 2008) requires the accrediting bodies of distance education programs to verify that the student taking the course is the student receiving credit for the work. Bailie and Jortberg (2009) describe the verification process with one university and an identity-verifying corporation.

Design consideration must be given to the level of assessment required for the course and the most appropriate method of assessment. If a paper or presentation can demonstrate that the student met the course objective, then perhaps testing is not necessary. Most CMSs have online testing capabilities that can be programmed for limited access, specific test-taking time, and random scrambling of test items and test answers. Using security, time limits, random delivery of test items, and scrambling of answer options assists in providing a measure of test security.

Proctored testing may be relevant for a high-stakes summative assessment, such as a graduation test, end-of-program exit exam and so on. Proctored testing at decentralized locations may be available to students at locations away from their own campuses. The Consortium of College Testing Centers (CCTC) is a free referral service provided by the National College Testing Association (2012). The CCTC consists of a group of 251 college and university testing centers throughout the United States that provides proctored testing at decentralized locations.

ADVANTAGES AND CHALLENGES OF TEACHING ONLINE FOR FACULTY

Some of the advantages of teaching online include flexibility and freedom from time constraints of the traditional classroom and the professional growth that occurs when faculty have the opportunity to move from lecturer and content expert to course facilitator using alternative forms of course delivery (Bristol, 2005; Johnson, Posey, & Simmens, 2005). Faculty also report that they have increased opportunity for rich interaction and discussions with students (Hurt, 2008). Reported challenges to teaching online include isolation and lack of face-to-face contact (Hurt, 2008) and increased workload (Ryan et al., 2004; Johnson et al., 2005; Manusco, 2009; Shelton & Saltsman, 2005).

Optimal class size is 20 to 25 students (Carlock, Hamrick, Johnson, Martell, & Schroeder, 2001). Some faculty report that the increased time required to develop and teach online courses is offset by the freedom and flexibility that come with teaching in this environment (Johnson, 2008). Also, once developed, the same course materials can be reused until revisions are needed. Once developed, the prep time needed is greatly reduced, which reduces faculty workload

SUMMARY AND KEY POINTS

Nursing education has experienced a paradigm shift with the introduction courses, curricula, and entire degree programs taught online. Many nurse educators have struggled with the change in teaching/learning environments and the technology. The transition to teaching online does not require that nursing faculty abandon the teaching methods and principles they have developed for traditional classroom instruction. The addition of online teaching strategies will complement a faculty's knowledge base and teaching abilities. This chapter discussed many of the issues that nursing faculty encounter when they make the transition from traditional classroom instruction to teaching online and offered a number of useful tools and resources to assist faculty.

REFERENCES

Acxiom. (2009). *Methods to verify the identity of distance learning students.* Retrieved from http://www.acxiom.com/SiteCollectionDocuments/website-resources/pdf/White_Papers/AC-0031-09_DistanceLearningStudentsWP.pdf

Alexander, J. W., Polyakova-Norwood, V., Johnston, L. W., Christensen, P., & Loquist, R. S. (2003). Collaborative development and evaluation of an online nursing course. *Distance Education, 24*(1), 41–56. doi:10.1080/01587910303046

Bailie, J. L., & Jortberg, M. A. (2009). Online learner authentication: Verifying the identity of online learners. *Journal of Online Learning and Teaching, 5*(2). Retrieved from http://jolt.merlot.org/vol5no2/bailie_0609.htm

Barczyk, C., Buckenmeyer, J., & Feldman, L. (2010). Mentoring professors: A model for developing quality online instructors and courses in higher education. *International Journal on E-Learning, 9*(1), 7–26.

Bates, A. W., & Poole, G. (2003). *Effective teaching with technology in higher education.* San Francisco, CA: Jossey-Bass.

Bristol, T. J. (2005). *Perceptions of e-learning in Iowa nursing faculty* (Doctoral dissertation). (UMI No. 3205702)

California State University, Chico. (2009). *Rubric for online instruction.* Retrieved from http://www.csuchico.edu/celt/roi/

Carlock, P., Hamrick, B., Johnson, C., Martell, K., & Schroeder, I. (2001). *Final report and recommendations: Faculty workload issues.* Retrieved from http://www.siue.edu/TLTR/GrpA4.htm

Cavanaugh, J. (2006). Comparing online time to offline time: The shocking truth. *Distance Education Report, 10*(9), 1–6.

Chickering, A. W., & Ehrmann, S. C. (1996). Implementing the seven principles: Technology as lever. *AAHE Bulletin.* Retrieved from http://www.wpi.edu/Academics/ATC/Collaboratory/Tips/General/principle1.html

Chickering, A. W., & Gamson, Z. F. (1987). Seven principles for good practice in undergraduate education. *AAHE Bulletin.* Retrieved from http://www.aahea.org/bulletins/articles/sevenprinciples1987.htm

Collison, G., Elbaum, B., Haavind, S., & Tinker, R. (2000). *Facilitating online learning: Effective strategies for moderators.* Madison, WI: Atwood Publishing.

Covington, D., Petherbridge, D., & Warren, S. E. (2005). Best practices: A triangulated support approach in transitioning faculty to online teaching. *Online Journal of Distance Learning Administration, 8*(1). Retrieved from http://www.westga.edu/~distance/ojdla/spring81/ covington81.htm

Cronenwett, L., Sherwood, G., Barnsteiner, J., Disch, J., Johnson, J., Mitchell, P., … Warren, J. (2007). Quality and safety education for nurses. Nursing Outlook, *55*(3), 122–131. doi:10.1016/j.outlook.2007.02.006

Edwards, M., Perry, B., & Janzen, K. (2011). The making of an exemplary online educator. *Distance Education, 32*(1), 101–118. doi:10.1080/01587919.2011.565499

Fehn, M. J. (2005). *An exploratory case study: Faculty perceptions of the barriers and obstacles to integrating web-based instruction into the associate degree nursing program* (Doctoral dissertation). (UMI No. 3179068)

Gallagher-Lepak, S., Reilly, J., & Killion, C. M. (2009). Nursing student perceptions of community in online learning. *Contemporary Nurse, 32*(1–2), 133–146.

Grant, M. R., & Thornton, H. R. (2007). Best practices in undergraduate adult-centered online learning: Mechanisms for course design and delivery. *Journal of Online Learning and Teaching, 3*(4), 346–356. Retrieved from http://jolt.merlot.org/documents/grant.pdf

Harasim, L. (1990). *On-line education: Perspectives on a new environment.* New York, NY: Praeger Publishers.

Hixon, E., & Zamojski, H. (2010, August). *The evolution of an online course development program.* Paper presented at the 26th Annual Conference on Distance Teaching & Learning, Madison, WI. Retrieved from http://www.uwex.edu/disted/conference/Resource_library/proceedings/29291_10.pdf

Holly, C., Legg, T. J., Mueller, D., & Adelman, D. S. (2008). Online teaching: Challenges for a new faculty role. *Journal of Professional Nursing, 24*(4), 254–258. doi:10.1016/j.profnurs.2007.07.003

Hudson Valley Community College. (n.d.). *HVCC guideline for best practices of online course design.* Retrieved from http://tlt.suny.edu/documentation/disted/HVCCbestpractices.pdf

Hurt, J. (2008). The advantages and disadvantages of teaching and learning online. *Delta Kappa Gamma Bulletin, 74*(4), 5–11.

Indiana University. (2011). *IT training & education*. Retrieved from http://ittraining.iu.edu/

Institute of Medicine. (2003). *Health professions education: A bridge to quality*. Washington, DC: The National Academies Press. Retrieved from http://www.iom.edu/Reports/2003/Health-Professions-Education-A-Bridge-to-Quality.aspx

Johnson, A. E. (2005). *Transition to online learning: The study of a graduate nursing faculty* (Doctoral dissertation). (UMI No. 3178470)

Johnson, A. E. (2008). A nursing faculty's transition to teaching online. *Nursing Education Perspectives, 29*(1), 17–22.

Johnson, J., Posey, L., & Simmens, S. J. (2005). Faculty and student perceptions of web-based learning: Bringing online educational programs to underserved communities. *American Journal for Nurse Practitioners, 9*(4), 9–18.

Keeton, M. T. (2004). Best online instruction practices: Report of phase I of an ongoing study. *Journal of Asynchronous Learning Networks, 8*(2), 75–100. Retrieved from http://sloanconsortium.org/jaln/v8n2/best-online-instructional-practices-report-phase-i-ongoing-study

Ko, S., & Rossen, S. (2010). *Teaching online. A practical guide* (3rd ed.). New York, NY: Routledge.

Koehler, M. J., Mishra, P. A., Hershey, K., & Peruski, L. (2004). With a little help from your students: A new model for faculty development and online course design. *Journal of Technology and Teacher Education, 12*(1), 25–55.

Kyrnin, J. (2012). *Are your web pages color sensitive?* About.com. Retrieved from http://webdesign.about.com/od/accessibility/a/aa062804.htm

Legg, T. J., Aldeman, D., & Levitt, C. (2009). Constructivist strategies in online distance education in nursing. *Journal of Nursing Education, 48*(2), 64–69.

Levin, J., Kim, H., & Riel. M. (1990) Analyzing instructional interactions on electronic message networks. In L. Harasim (Ed.), *Online education: Perspectives on a new environment* (pp. 185-214). New York, NY: Praeger Publishers.

Long, K. A. (2003). The Institute of Medicine report: Health professions education: A bridge to quality. *Policy, Politics, & Nursing Practice, 4*(4), 259–262. doi:10.1177/1527154403258304

Lunney, M., & Sammarco, A. (2009). Scoring rubric for grading students' participation in online discussions. *CIN: Computers, Informatics, Nursing, 27*(1), 26–31. doi:10.1097/NCN.0b013e31818dd3f6

Lynch, M. (2002). *The online educator: A guide to creating the virtual classroom*. New York, NY: Routledge. doi:10.4324/9780203458556

Macy, R. (2007). The transition from face-to-face to online teaching. *Campus Technology 2007*. Retrieved from http://download.101com.com/CAM/conf/2007/Macy.pdf

Manusco, J. M. (2009). Perceptions of distance education among nursing faculty members in North America. *Nursing and Health Sciences, 11*(2), 194–205. doi:10.1111/j.1442-2018.2009.00456.x

Mastrian, K. G., McGonigle, D., Mahan, W. L., & Bixler, B. (2011). *Integrating technology in nursing education. Tools for the knowledge era*. Sudbury, MA: Jones and Bartlett Publishers.

Mayne, L. A., & Wu, Q. (2011). Creating and measuring social presence in online graduate nursing courses. *Nursing Education Perspectives, 32*(2), 110–114. doi:10.5480/1536-5026-32.2.110

Moore, G. S., Winograd, K., & Lange, D. (2001). *You can teach online: Building a creative learning environment*. New York, NY: McGraw-Hill.

National College Testing Association. (2012). About the consortium. Retrieved from http://www.ncta-testing.org/cctc/

Online Teaching Resources. (2011). *Technical prerequisite skills checklist*. Retrieved from http://www.sanjuancollege.edu/pages/2848.asp

Palloff, R. M., & Pratt, K. (2003). *The virtual student: A profile and guide to working with online learners.* San Francisco, CA: Jossey-Bass.

Palloff, R. M., & Pratt, K. (2011). *The excellent online instructors. Strategies for professional development.* San Francisco, CA: Jossey-Bass.

Pankowski, P. (2004). Faculty training for online teaching. *T.H.E. Journal.* Retrieved from http://thejournal.com/Articles/2004/09/01/Faculty-Training-for-Online-Teaching.aspx#

Paradise Community College. (n.d.). *Is online teaching for me?* Retrieved from http://www2.pvc.maricopa.edu/~fog/isonlineforme.html

Pennsylvania State University. (2009). *Faculty self assessment for online teaching.* Retrieved from http://weblearning.psu.edu/news/faculty-self-assessment

Perreault, H., Waldman, L., Alexander, M., & Zhao, J. (2008). Comparing the distance learning-related course development approach and faculty support and rewards structure at AACSB accredited institutions between 2001 and 2006. *The Journal of Educators Online, 5*(2). Retrieved from http://www.thejeo.com/Volume5Number2/PerreaultetalPaper.pdf

Robina, K. A., & Anderson, M. L. (2010). Online teaching efficacy of nursing faculty. *Journal of Professional Nursing, 26*(3), 168–175. doi:10.1016/j.profnurs.2010.02.006

Rowe, N. C. (2004). Cheating in online student assessment: Beyond plagiarism. *Online Journal of Distance Learning Administration, 7*(2). Retrieved from http://www.westga.edu/ ~distance/ojdla/summer72/rowe72.html

Ryan, M., Carlton, K., & Ali, N. S. (2004). Role of faculty in distance learning and changing pedagogies. *Nursing Education Perspectives, 25*(2), 73–80.

Savery, J. R., & Duffy, T. M. (2006). Problem based learning: An instructional model and its constructivist framework. In B. Wilson (Ed.), *Constructivist learning environments: Case studies in instructional design.* Englewood Cliffs, NJ: Educational Technology.

Sewell, J. P., Frith, K. H., & Colvin, M. M. (2010). Online assessment strategies: A primer. *Journal of Online Learning and Teaching, 6*(1). 297–305. Retrieved from http://jolt.merlot.org/vol6no1/sewell_0310.pdf

Shea, P., Fredericksen, E., Pickett, A., & Pelz, W. (2003). *A preliminary investigation of teaching presence in the SUNY learning network, elements of quality online education.* Needham, MA: SCOLE.

Shelton, K., & Saltsman, G. (2005). *An administrator's guide to online education.* Greenwich, CT: Information Age Publishing.

Skiba, D., & Barton, A. (2006). Adapting your teaching to accommodate the net generation of learners. *The Online Journal of Issues in Nursing, 11*(2). Retrieved from http://www.nursingworld.org/MainMenuCategories/ANAMarketplace/ANAPeriodicals/OJIN/TableofContents/Volume112006/No2May06/tpc30_416076.aspx

Sunal, D., Hodges, J., Sunal, C., Whitaker, K., Freeman, L., Edwards L., … Odell, M. (2001). Teaching science in higher education: Faculty professional development and barriers to change. *School Science and Mathematics, 101*(5), 246-257. doi:10.1111/j.1949-8594.2001.tb18027.x

Swan, K., Shen, J., & Hiltz, S. R. (2006). Assessment and collaboration in online learning. *Journal of Asynchronous Learning Networks, 10*(1), 45–62. Retrieved from http://www-new.kent.edu/ehhs/dl/upload/assessment-and-collaboration.pdf

Taylor, A., & McQuiggan, C. (2008). Faculty development programming: If we build it, will they come? *EDUCAUSE Quarterly, 31*(3), 29–37. Retrieved from http://connect.educause.edu/Library/EDUCAUSE+Quarterly/EDUCAUSEQuarterlyMagazine/47096

Taylor, J. (2003). Managing staff development for online education: A situated learning model. *Journal of Higher Education Policy and Management, 25*(1), 75–87. doi:10.1080/1360080032000067013

Teaching Styles Quiz. (2001). *Teaching styles self evaluation.* Retrieved from http://members.shaw.ca/mdde615/tchstylsquiz7.htm

Thurmond, V., & Wambach, K. (2004). Understanding interactions in distance education: A review of the literature. *International Journal of Instructional Technology & Distance Learning*. Retrieved from http://www.itdl.org/journal/jan_04/article02.htm

UDI Online provides faculty with e-tools to increase accessibility of online courses. (2011). *Disability Compliance for Higher Education, 16*(10), 4–5. doi:10.1002/dhe.20041

United States Department of Education. (2008). *Higher Education Opportunity Act*. Retrieved from http://www2.ed.gov/policy/highered/leg/hea08/index.html

Universal Design Education. (n.d.). University at Buffalo. Retrieved from http://www.udeducation.org/

University of Arkansas at Little Rock. (2010). *Online education*. Retrieved from http://ualr.edu/pace/index.php/home/hot-topics/online-ed/

University of Birmingham. (2012). *Learning development unit*. Retrieved from http://www.ldu.bham.ac.uk/elearn/

Wisconsin Online. (2011). *Learning objects*. Retrieved from http://www.wisconline.com/listobjects.aspx

Worley, W. L., & Tesdell, L. S. (2009). Instructor time and effort in online and face-to-face teaching: Lessons learned. *IEEE Transactions on Professional Communication, 52*(2), 138–151. Retrieved from https://collab.cosolvent.com/ccs/main.php?g2_view=core.DownloadItem&g2_itemId=2046&g2_dl=0

Zsohar, H., & Smith, J. A. (2008). Transition from the classroom to the web: Successful strategies for teaching online. *Nursing Education Perspectives, 29*(1), 23–28.

FOUR

Exemplars of Faculty Preparation

DEBORAH J. CLARK

Most nurse educators who teach online have learning needs. The gaps in knowledge vary based on past teaching experience and computer skills. Even nurse educators who have taught online for many years have professional development needs because technology changes so rapidly. In order to understand faculty preparation, three experienced nurse educators were interviewed about their current professional work, the process of learning to use distance education, unique opportunities at their universities, their evaluation methods in online courses, and advice they would give a new nurse educator. These nurse educators teach in RN-BSN, master's, and doctoral programs. They generously gave of their time and expertise to this chapter.

RN-BSN DISTANCE EDUCATION: Flor Culpa-Bondal, PhD, RN

Dr. Culpa-Bondal is an assistant professor at Georgia College & State University (GC&SU), Milledgeville, Georgia, in the College of Health Sciences. She has been employed by the university for 9 years and has more than 11 years of teaching experience. She is a graduate of Holy Name University in the Philippines and has a master's in nursing and a post-master's in nursing informatics from GC&SU. Her PhD is from Texas Woman's University. Dr. Culpa-Bondal was an online student in her post-master's informatics program and in the PhD program. The PhD program used a hybrid format with class meetings only monthly during the semester. Her teaching experience in the RN-BSN program includes the courses Transitions to Baccalaureate Nursing and the Research in Professional Practice.

Dr. Culpa-Bondal's personal interest in distance education began during the doctoral program. The courses offered an autonomous, facilitated but self-directed learning environment. This form of learning was transformative for her and provided the liberty of choosing a quality education at a distance from her home without needing to physically attend classes each week.

Beginning to Teach Online

Nursing faculty, beginning back in the late 1990s, were some of the most innovative early adopters of online education in the university. Faculty support for online education on the GC&SU campus was fashioned initially after the University System of Georgia's Faculty Development Boot Camp started in 1995. Faculty from across the university who had attended this 2-week intensive workshop returned to campus to develop and lead the workshop at the GC&SU campus. From the outset, GC&SU's workshop was designed to focus first on pedagogy and second on instructional technology. Later, this group formally established the Center for Excellence in Teaching and Learning (CETL, www.gcsu.edu/cetl). Each year, two faculty members volunteered to chair and cochair CETL. Deans granted these faculty members a one-course release for their leadership roles. The Director of Information and Instructional Technology arranged for funding of CETL to provide incentives for faculty participation such as laptop computers, personal digital assistants (PDAs), and equipment for podcasting. The CETL planned the curriculum of programs and purchased books for faculty to support their development. CETL remains a faculty-driven organization guided by a steering committee comprised of faculty members from across the university.

When a learning management system (LMS) was adopted, a new department in the university was formed, called Web Enabled Resources (WER), which was staffed by instructional technology specialists. WER provided services such as the on-campus LMS training, online training modules, podcasting, website design, and other projects (WER website, www.gcsu.edu/library/wer/index.htm; GC&SU, 2011). WER continues to provide faculty with updates on the changes in the LMS and assists students and faculty with troubleshooting problems.

Dr. Culpa Bondal's initial orientation to online teaching came through GC&SU's CETL. Because Dr. Culpa Bondal was an experienced teacher, her professional development focused on designing multimedia content to achieve learning outcomes and developing assessments to measure learning gains. Other faculty in the College of Health Sciences who needed different professional development attended the CETL workshop and worked one-on-one with a faculty expert in curriculum design. Because nearly all of the nursing faculty members attended CETL's online teaching workshops, excitement for distance education was present, and the resources needed to be successful were available.

The School of Nursing currently offers face-to-face, hybrid, and online courses across the curriculum. Faculty with experience in distance education support new and current faculty with the development of skills and abilities needed to teach nursing at a distance or in a classroom. Topics covered in faculty education include principles of adult learning, curriculum design, and methods of assessing learning from a distance.

Process of Learning to Teach the First Course

For Dr. Culpa-Bondal, teaching online was chaotic at first. She began with simply taking her traditional classroom materials and placing them online. She posted the syllabus, calendar, and other materials there for students to view and use. At first, she did not use a course orientation, but now she has a fully developed orientation to her course. The course orientation includes a module provided by WER, which covers how to send and receive e-mail, how to submit an assignment, taking tests, and posting questions in the forum. In addition to the orientation, students take the Kingdomality® Personal Preference Profile test (www.cmi-lmi.com/kingdom.html) and post an introduction of themselves in a discussion forum. The Kingdomality test is given as an icebreaker, but she uses the personality types to form working groups within the class.

Dr. Culpa-Bondal became confident in her abilities once she could anticipate the issues commonly seen in the LMS, design of the course, and course content in general. Some things cannot be controlled in the online environment, so knowing and accepting this makes it easier to teach online. In face-to-face class settings, students can ask their questions and have an immediate answer. The online environment seems to be immediate, but in reality, time can be taken to formulate answers to student e-mails and responses to student posts. Dr. Culpa-Bondal wishes she could give each student immediate feedback but knows this is not realistic because she is not online in the classroom 24/7 to answer questions.

She describes herself as a competent online instructor. The courses she develops now use most features of the LMS including grading forms, announcements, and blogs, and she has more experience in developing classes for the online environment. In the past year, the RN-BSN program was revised to take full advantage of online pedagogy. The learning activities in each course were designed to make full use of the LMS, for example, SoftChalk™ (softchalk.com) for lessons compatible with mobile devices and LiveText™ (www.livetext.com) e-portfolios are used.

Evaluating Teaching and Learning

For Dr. Culpa-Bondal, the one activity that supported a clearer view of the curriculum evaluation process has been mapping learning outcomes to learning assessments and evaluation. The mapping was done when the course was first designed, and the assessment results are reviewed during and at the end of the semester. She sets benchmarks for achievement of the learning outcomes and compares these to the evaluation results. These data are then used to improve the course for the next time it is offered. She also asks the students for their feedback on whether or not an activity was effective.

One example of using student feedback to improve a course was described by Dr. Culpa-Bondal. When first teaching, each week's learning module was revealed ("opened") to students, discussed, and closed in a week's time. The students felt rushed and complained about how overwhelming the pace of the course was. Now, she organizes her courses with 1 week of content, then a discussion week, then a week of content, and another discussion week. She finds this pace more relaxed but also a more robust teaching–learning experience, and the outcomes are good.

Maintaining Online/Distance Education Teaching Skills

When asked about the activities she engages in to develop or maintain her teaching skills, Dr. Culpa-Bondal has many. She subscribes to Faculty Focus (www.facultyfocus.com) and reads their articles and reports. She attends CETL conferences university-wide and in the University System of Georgia. She and her husband have a CNET (www.cnet.com) subscription that keeps them up-to-date with technology.

The College of Health Sciences and the nursing faculty support online teaching and the use of technology. When new tools and software come to the marketplace, faculty requests for purchase are almost always supported. Nursing faculty are encouraged to attend the Faculty Development Workshop and can negotiate their teaching hours so they can attend.

Future of Distance Education in Nursing

The future will bring new technology and unique ways of working with information where the student can manipulate charts, pictures, tables, and information wirelessly and using voice. Dr. Culpa-Bondal believes that online classrooms will be more affordable, portable, and accessible. The capabilities of technology make both synchronous and asynchronous features a way to improve the students' abilities to interact with faculty, peers, and course content. The teacher's challenge will be staying current with the changing technology and maintaining current materials and assessments.

Selected Distance Education Activities That Demonstrate Recommendations From the Carnegie Report

One activity that supports the recommendation to "shift from an emphasis on socialization and role-taking to an emphasis on formation" (Benner, Stuphen, Leonard, & Day, 2009) is described by Dr. Culpa-Bondal. She sees the former RN-BSN students as beginning the program without seeing the added value of the program outcomes to their careers. When the RN-BSN program moved from the traditional setting to the online setting, the curriculum and pedagogies aligned to distance education. Using a mentorship model, students are asked to state their career goals in alignment with the program outcomes. Having career goals that align with the education program's outcomes can signify that the student is in the right program. A mentor can then be selected to match the student's career goals and support the educational experience. Since the courses' outcomes are aligned with the program outcomes, it could be said that courses should help graduates achieve their career goals. The mentorship model is carried throughout the courses, with planned activities for the mentor–mentee dyads. As students progress, they develop an e-portfolio of evidence that supports each of the program outcomes. This "formation" is individualized and thus more meaningful to the student.

PhD IN A NURSING DISTANCE EDUCATION PROGRAM: Judith A. Effken, PhD, RN, FACMI, FAAN

Dr. Effken taught online for 10 years at the University of Arizona College of Nursing, where she is professor emerita and adjunct research professor. She holds a BA in psychology from the University of Hartford and an MS in nursing management and a PhD in psychology with a focus on cognition and instruction from the University of Connecticut. Her personal interest in distance education coincided with the College of Nursing's motivation to make its PhD program available online so that more nurses had access to the university. At first, the program considered telemedicine technology but ruled that out because it did not offer access to students outside Arizona. Providing an online curriculum offered broader access to the University and an opportunity to make the doctoral courses more interactive.

The PhD in Nursing and the Doctor of Nursing Practice (DNP) programs are delivered in an online format (www.nursing.arizona.edu) using Desire2Learn™ (www.desire2learn.com). Dr. Effken has taught health care informatics, theory and practice, health care data management, and technology for enhancing health care delivery online. She has experience teaching in a variety of nursing programs including PhD, DNP, and master's degree students from a variety of disciplines, although she has never been an online student herself.

Developing the Online Doctoral Program

Initially, the nursing faculty held a retreat where the program values and goals for the online doctorate were discussed. The faculty discussed what they valued and thus what they wanted to retain and change in the doctoral program. As a result, a handbook was written to guide the implementation of the online doctoral program and proved useful during the process. Several books related to teaching online were purchased for faculty reference. Faculty were oriented to online teaching through a university program that was combined with a day spent with Dr. Diane Skiba from the University of Colorado and Dr. Rick Zoucha from Duquesne University. This one-on-one faculty contact helped the program faculty members understand the possibilities in online education as well as allay fears about how particular content could be taught in the online environment.

Work by faculty was supported directly and indirectly by two grants. The first provided for course release or supplemental compensation over the summer for course design. The second supported the university's technology team. As the project chair, Dr. Effken supported the faculty and designed her own course. Brown-bag sessions during the course development period helped faculty share their successes and experiences.

Although there currently is no formal training in online education available to faculty, the university offers a variety of courses in adult learning, curriculum design, and evaluation. Dr. Effken believes that the ideal method for orienting faculty to online teaching is to gain their buy-in first (e.g., through the retreat) instead of having the decision made by others to change an in-seat program to an online program. Consultants helped faculty envision how they might revise their courses into terrific online classes that meet the students' needs as well as the program outcomes. Having an instructional designer and technical support staff was crucial so the faculty could concentrate on the pedagogy (and not so much the technology). She recommends that a faculty member who designs an online course teach it at least three times in order to evaluate the design and outcomes before other faculty teach the course.

Process of Learning to Teach the First Course

Dr. Effken developed her first course over one semester and had the entire course available to learners on the first day. The course contained mini lectures in PowerPoint format that provided an overview of each module. Self-quizzes for self-knowledge checks were included in the course. Students worked on real-world individual and group projects that kept them actively involved in the course content.

A primary learning activity was group discussions, which can be one of the more challenging aspects of teaching online. Dr. Effken posted a grading rubric and provided guidelines for the discussions, which comprised 20% of the course grade. She reported that finding the right amount of interaction in group discussions is a learned skill that comes with practice. Learning from experience and experts, Dr. Effken believes that it is more effective for instructors to monitor the discussion, encourage students to build on each other's ideas, challenge students to think critically about the topics, and intervene if the discussion takes a wrong turn. The program faculty found that with the online discussions, at all levels of education (MSN, doctoral), students discussed course topics at a higher level. Because the discussions were asynchronous, all students could carefully consider their responses before posting. This contrasts with the traditional classroom setting where students who can think on their feet may dominate discussions. During student orientation, students are given useful tools to manage group work. Admittedly, some students do not embrace group work.

The time commitment for teaching online varies with the faculty member, but Dr. Effken believes the faculty should agree on the standards so that students see consistency among the faculty. Group assignments are always challenging. Dr. Effken relates that the faculty have tried numerous methods to form groups, including self-selection and random assignment. With large class sizes, managing groups is a priority for faculty and students. Although most discussions are asynchronous, some discussions do occur synchronously. Dr. Effken always holds a final synchronous online discussion related to the final class projects. The date and time of the discussion is posted in the syllabus. Students post an executive summary and a narrated PowerPoint for their classmates prior to the discussion. The class discusses the projects and asks questions of each group. These final discussions are so popular that she often has to tell her students to "go home" when the class time runs out.

Designing Courses Now

Dr. Effken uses constructivist theories, including the ecological approach to instructional design (Effken et al., 2009). The Community of Inquiry (COI) model (fostering cognitive presence, social presence, and teaching presence) is also used in the doctoral program. Dr. Effken finds the COI model ideal for the doctoral program. The program also holds a weeklong Resident Intensive Summer Experience (RISE) for doctoral students (www.nursing.arizona.edu/RISE.htm). The program covers expectations for doctoral study, the online learning experience, and some of the courses. In addition, this face-to-face time with students is used to simulate real-world experiences that are better done in person.

Dr. Effken has used Elluminate®, Skype®, and Audacity®. E-activities encourage students to go online to discover or find new information that is reported back to the group discussions. She finds that it is best to decide, as a faculty member, which tools will be used and to limit the number so that students do not need to learn too many.

The biggest change Dr. Effken experienced was a dramatic rise in the number of enrollments in her primary course. Accommodating a larger number of students within one course section required dividing the class into separate groups. Also, students entering the class directly from a BSN program required more detailed information in the syllabus.

Evaluation of Teaching and Learning

Dr. Effken uses her own observations and students' feedback to incorporate changes into her courses annually. When the number of BS-DNP students enrolled in her informatics course increased, structured support for students through a more detailed syllabus was needed. She recommends that faculty use midcourse evaluations; the university's teaching/learning student evaluations, with additional questions for students related to the specific technologies used in the class; and peer evaluation of the course during and after course design. Having external evaluation by a peer or other expert adds to the validation process. Dr. Effken strongly recommends that faculty adopt a teaching–learning model as the basis for development and assessment of the program.

The College of Nursing uses several evaluation tools. A general evaluation tool was developed by a former University of Alabama faculty member who specialized in evaluation. The program also used the University of Arizona course/faculty evaluation of instruction and a third special evaluation developed by the instructional designer aimed at evaluating the technology used in the course. At one point, the college invited Dr. Diane Billings, an expert in online teaching and learning, to evaluate the courses. From the instructor perspective, midcourse evaluations were used to assess student progress so that changes could be made during the class if needed.

Maintaining Online/Distance Education Teaching Skills

To maintain her online teaching skills, Dr. Effken attends and/or presents at her university's annual instructional technology day and several educational conferences and reads widely, particularly about discussions and e-activities. She has been involved in developing sets of courses in tandem with other professors. The University of Arizona's Master's Entry to the Profession of Nursing (MEPN) program (initial licensure program for nurses with a prior bachelor's degree in another field) has three such courses where a major project is built across the span of three classes. In the doctoral program, larger modules that span 2 to 3 weeks provide students time to prepare themselves before participating in discussions. She is interested in evaluation of the larger classes, particularly in assessing the group outcomes, processes, and individual contributions within groups.

Future of Online Teaching

Dr. Effken believes that although online teaching is growing rapidly, not all programs are preparing and supporting nursing faculty well. Online courses are not the same as the in-seat versions and often require as much, if not more, faculty time for planning, developing, and evaluating the courses. Most PhD programs are relatively small. As a result, faculty expertise in any one program is limited. To share expertise, several consortia-based programs have developed, including the consortium among Big 10 universities and NEXus, a program among Western universities. These programs can offer students access to greater variety in courses and faculty. Dr. Effken hopes that more doctoral programs will work together to eliminate the barriers to forming consortia, such as fee differentials and administrative red tape.

Faculty must own the online program, according to Dr. Effken. Technology support is essential, including instructional designers who help ensure consistency of design across the program and hold the hands of faculty during the development process. Paying faculty for their redesign time is essential. Recognition for creativity, successful design, and online teaching in the annual evaluation process is also important.

Pearls of Wisdom From Our Experts

- Start with good course design. Work backward in design by beginning with what you want the outcomes to be. Design activities and assignments to meet the outcomes given the time, tools, and educational materials available
- Provide clear instructions in all parts of your course—but particularly the syllabus
- Spend time learning how to facilitate discussions because it is a major learning activity in an online course
- When working with groups, remember that they go through the same group formation milestones that face-to-face groups experience, so prepare students to manage the stages of group formation
- Experiencing an online class yourself can provide opportunities to see what works and what does not work well
- Learn to use the LMS's tools by playing and experimenting. Once you know what is available, you can be more creative with the assignments and other learning activities
- Join online discussion forums for your selected LMS to expand what you know and your problem-solving skills
- Set a schedule to go into your online classroom often. Some students will check the course daily, while others may need a helpful reminder to "attend" class. Find a happy balance for all

participants. Let your students know how often you will be in the classroom and when they can expect feedback on assignments

- Have one design and appearance for all the online classrooms. This prevents students from having to relearn the layout of the classroom. Keep it simple and uncluttered
- The fewer "clicks," the better. Navigation should also be simple and quick

REFERENCE

Effken, J., McEwen, M. Vincent, D., Shea, K., Garcia-Smith, D., Kang, Y., & Young, M. (2009). Application and evaluation of the ecological psychology approach to instructional design (EPAID). *Journal of Asynchronous Learning Networks, 13*(4), 41–56. Retrieved from http://sloanconsortium.org/jaln/v13n4/application-and-evaluation-ecological-psychology-approach-instructional-design-epaid

FIVE

Supporting Learner Success

SUSAN ALEXANDER and HALEY HOY

One role of the distance education (DE) instructor is to assist students, many of whom are used to learning in a traditional classroom, in becoming successful distance learners. Learning how to support nursing students in a DE program involves knowing the special barriers and challenges of being a successful online learner. In this chapter, specific factors critical to the support of the DE learner include assessing learner motivation, readiness, enabling factors, and barriers to success. Informing and orienting learners to the DE environment, providing technical support, and offering the same campus resources to DE students as in-seat students are additional success factors for nursing students. Finally, providing opportunities to build the one-on-one connections between learner and teacher, learner and content, and learners with peers builds relationships that support learner success.

LEARNER MOTIVATIONS IN DISTANCE EDUCATION COURSES

Reasons for Taking Online Courses

Flexibility in scheduling and geographic location, access to nursing education, and cost savings are the three main reasons for choosing an online learning format over the traditional classroom (Braun, 2008; Moskal & Dziuban, 2001; Parsad & Lewis, 2008). A student's ability to complete coursework on a personal schedule that does not conflict with work or family responsibilities creates an opportunity for continuing formal education (Stanford-Bowers, 2008). Flexibility applies to providing convenient meeting spaces, classroom materials, and learning opportunities, as well as access to expert faculty in distant physical locations. Students who live at a distance from campus can attend courses not traditionally taught locally and with expert faculty. DE programs can help create partnerships that would not otherwise be possible (American Association of Colleges of Nursing [AACN], 2011). In fact, student access to college in general, especially in rural areas, is achievable through DE (Parsad & Lewis, 2008).

Financial issues related to DE remain a primary reason students take online courses. Depending on the type of institution (private or public), tuition can be affordable, particularly if students can continue to work (Holly, 2009). Cost avoidance is also a benefit because students can avoid the cost of a commute to campus, the need for child care, and high costs of textbooks by using e-books or teacher-supplied online materials (Moskal & Dziuban, 2001; Parsad & Lewis, 2008). However, expenses such as out-of-state tuition, technology fees, and start-up technology such as a computer, required software, and Internet access may offset some of the cost savings.

Learner Readiness

Assessing learner readiness is a key component to success in teaching, regardless of the format. This step can mean the difference between course frustration and student/teacher satisfaction (Watkins, Leigh, & Triner, 2004). In a traditional classroom, learner readiness is generally observed with facial expression and open-discussion question-and-answer sessions (Marshall & Drummond, 2006). In DE programs, it may be technically difficult or impossible to assess facial expressions. Therefore, there is an additional need to assess technological capacity, skill, and motivation before beginning an online class or program. DE programs conduct assessments of DE student readiness by simple surveys of the type of computer hardware and software owned, ability to use the Internet, and learning styles (Parkland College, 2011; Pennsylvania State University, 2011; University of Houston Distance Education, 2011). The schools (and students) use the results of such surveys to determine the suitability of online education for individual learners.

With DE, both synchronous and asynchronous interactions between instructors and students provide an opportunity to assess readiness and skills. With DE courses, instructors can assess aspects of technological capability and skill by evaluating the student's ability to interact with course materials, peers, and the instructor. Initial comfort and level of knowledge of the subject matter can be seen in timely, well-developed responses to discussion questions and replies to peers. In asynchronous discussions, students are allowed to contribute as much as they would like to in a given discussion, often with the expectations for interaction defined by the instructor (Gallogly, 2005). An assessment of the level and depth of a discussion response, and timeliness, can reflect student knowledge and ability to navigate the online classroom and course materials.

Enabling Factors for Online Learning

With dropout rates in DE as high as 30% to 50%, understanding persistence of students in DE courses is critical (Stanford-Bowers, 2008). Kember's model of student persistence in a course includes factors affecting working adult learners such as entry characteristics (age, years worked, gender, marital status, salary, educational background); social integration compared to external attribution; academic incompatibility compared to academic integration; grade point average (GPA); and cost–benefit analysis. If students stay on a positive path, they are likely to persist in their programs. If students stay on a negative path, they are likely to drop out or leave their programs (McGivny, 2009). Certainly DE students are challenged by family life, work, and other issues that compete for their time and attention.

In order to understand the perceptions of persistence by students, faculty, and administrators in DE courses, Stanford-Bowers (2008) conducted a Delphi study to find the top 10 factors. Only three enabling factors were common to the three groups: time management, having clearly stated requirements, and computer access. Students reported that the most important enabling factors were convenience and flexibility of DE classes, having good time-management skills, and having clearly stated course requirements. Teachers perceived that self-motivation of students, clearly stated course requirements, and responsiveness of the teacher were the most important enabling factors. Administrators believed that self-discipline of students, responsiveness of the teacher, and self-motivation of students were critical to enable DE persistence.

Persistence in DE courses has also been linked to internal locus of control (Parker, 2003). Not only were students who had an internal locus of control more persistent, but they also showed a statistically significant increase in internal locus of control when comparing measurements at the beginning of the course to the end of the course. DE faculty actions taken to improve persistence include having a high quantity and quality of interactions with the students, showing responsiveness to the needs and questions of DE learners, and providing clear instructions in all areas of the DE course.

Barriers to Online Learning

Barriers to online learning for students include a lack of essential computer equipment, poor computer skills, and the feeling of social isolation in DE programs (Carruth, Broussard, Waldmeier, Gauthier, & Mixon, 2010). Technical requirements include hardware, software, and Internet access. Start-up cost for a student with no basic computer access can be large (typically over $800). In addition, there can be additional costs for course-related software and Internet service. Some of these expenses are offset by a savings in travel expense, but not all. Social isolation and a sense of alienation have been reported by students new to online education, particularly in courses not designed to encourage interaction (Fahy & Ally, 2005; Gallogly, 2005; Hammond, 2005).

INFORMING THE LEARNER ABOUT COURSES

The convenience and ease of access offered by DE can be attractive for students, but the reality is that the coursework is often more challenging when compared to a traditional classroom, particularly when the necessity of technical skills is considered. The student who is interested in these programs should be aware of the limited face-to-face contact between instructor and student and the need for self-direction and autonomy. In discussing educational programs with prospective students, marketing representatives for colleges and universities should provide clear descriptions of differences between online and traditional classrooms. The placement of demonstration class modules or tutorials on institutional websites can serve as a trial run in the pre-enrollment phase.

ORIENTING LEARNERS TO DISTANCE EDUCATION

Once a student has made the decision to enroll in a DE program, orientation should take place quickly and include specific requirements regarding technology, program expectations, and roles for the successful student. The use of standardized orientation programs that students can access after registration help to better prepare students for coursework (Billings, 2000). The Western Interstate Commission for Higher Education (WICHE) Center for Educational Technology (2001) recommended, in its best practices for institutions offering degree and certificate programs online, that students be informed about required access to technology and minimum technical competence prior to enrolling in an online course. Frith and Kee (2003) suggested that initial orientation sessions for DE courses be conducted in a face-to-face session whenever possible and should provide a list of technical criteria designed to screen out students who may be unable to participate due to a lack of computer skills. Other authors support the need for precourse orientation and assessment of technical skills, notification of hardware and software requirements, and participation in orientation to online courses well in advance of course start dates (Atack & Rankin, 2002) for prospective students and novice learners. Jenkins (2011) takes the idea one step further by suggesting that students should take a 1-hour course for credit to prepare them for the learner-centered approach used in DE and to bolster technical skills.

Technology

Interaction with a web-based learning system should be a comfortable experience and not serve as a physical or functional barrier to the use of DE programs (Bouhnik & Marcus, 2006). Because issues of incompatibility and interoperability may be difficult for even the most seasoned computer user, faculty and support staff should assist learners in managing frustrating technical difficulties. With the increasing availability of broadband access, learning management systems (LMS) are robust and can support all types of multimedia. It is common for the LMS to require installation of plug-ins or add-ons for the student to experience complete functionality of the system. Lists of these requirements, along with other system tests, should be visible on the log-in page for an LMS. Browser compatibility with an LMS and its components may vary throughout the student's experience in DE programs, as newer software versions may not be supported by the LMS or its components.

Expectations

Students who enroll in DE programs should be advised about the amount of time they can expect to spend in class participation and preparation. On a weekly basis, undergraduate students typically spend 2 hours per course credit hour in study and preparation. Graduate students might spend 3 hours per course credit hour weekly in similar activities. Online students who are performing the bulk of reading, studying, and assignment preparation may require more time.

To underscore the need for student engagement, faculty members must be clear about criteria for student participation in courses. For example, the use of discussion forums can serve as a means of increasing student–student interaction, fostering a sense of community along the way. By providing clear instructions regarding minimum requirements for the quality, time frame, and length of postings to discussion forums, instructors can assist students in both prioritizing and preparing assignments. Providing a list of guidelines for netiquette within the course framework can help students to understand the role of a course member.

Roles

The need for active participation in online coursework cannot be overemphasized; students must accept responsibility for their learning experience (Allen & Seaman, 2005). Students who are most successful in DE programs are highly self-regulated and autonomous, with the ability to prioritize assignments and better-than-average time-management skills (Barnard-Brak, Lon, & Paton, 2010). Sung (2006) further described five attributes that are predictive of academic success in DE: "intrinsic goal orientation (motivation), Internet self-efficacy, time management, study environment management, and learning assistance management (help-seeking)" (pp. 41–43). Initiative, persistence, and resourcefulness are necessary characteristics for the autonomous learner (Confessore & Park, 2004).

Early instructor intervention regarding time management is crucial to student success in online learning. Particularly when students are new to online classes, fear of failure and a lack of time-management skills can derail the even the most well-intended student.

Special Needs

Institutions of higher education that offer DE have a responsibility to make online learning accessible for students with special needs. Section 508 is an amendment to the Workforce Rehabilitation Act of 1973 that describes standards for ensuring that a website or class is accessible for people with disabilities (United States Access Board, 2011). Subpart B of the standards includes guidelines for software applications and operating systems; web intranet and Internet information and applications; telecommunications products; self-contained, closed products; and desktop and portable computers. Subpart C covers functional performance criteria for those with impaired vision, hearing, speech, or fine motor control. Features that improve the DE experience for students with special needs include the use of speech recognition software and audio files for lecture materials for visually impaired students. Features such as keyboard navigation commands in lieu of mouse manipulation for those students with impaired mobility are also available.

Students with non-English-speaking backgrounds (NESBs) comprise another group of students who may have difficulty with course success when compared to those speaking English as a primary language. In his analysis of reasons for failure in DE learners, Rolfe (2007) found that faculty members were ". . . not equipped to teaching students who did not have proficiency in the English language" (p. 12). In a comparison of late submissions for online and traditional assignments from 2003 to 2006, 25% of online students submitted assignments late compared to 5% of traditional students. The primary cause for the late submissions was the difficulty of ESL (English as a second language) students in understanding instructions for submission (Rolfe, 2007).

PROVIDING TECHNICAL SUPPORT

According to the AACN (2011), nursing students ". . . are usually quite willing to attempt new approaches to learning, but have little patience with ineffective or unreliable technologies." Although costly, 24/7 technical support is necessary for student retention in DE programs by phone, e-mail, or online chat. A list of designated staff or faculty, along with rapid contact information, should be available to students upon registration to classes and posted on the institution's LMS home page. Issues concerning access to the LMS or the functionality of its components should be resolved as quickly as possible to maintain or increase student satisfaction (Bouhnik & Marcus, 2006). DE instructors are also providers of technical support and are responsible for some of the functionality of the course.

Hardware and Software

Due to the variability in hardware requirements for LMS, institutions should maintain updated lists of needs for their system of choice. Specifications should include type of operating system, memory, processor speed, necessary bandwidth, hard-drive space, and minimum display resolution. Software requirements in DE program courses should focus on the use of common applications, such as word processing, spreadsheets, and presentation software. Programs such as these are in wide use, and most software providers have online tutorials, movies, or user manuals that help students to find answers when questions arise. Student versions of software programs can also decrease costs. OpenOffice™ (www.openoffice.org) is an example of a free word processing resource.

In addition, compatibility issues between operating systems, software applications, and the LMS may create fewer problems for students when common applications are used. Specificity in requirements of file submission for assignments should be established at the beginning of each course, allowing students who may be less familiar with applications an opportunity to practice their skills. Unfamiliarity with the use of software applications may increase the time necessary to prepare and submit assignments. In surveying cumulative data from a group of 24 colleges, Rolfe (2007) identified unfamiliarity with use of software applications as a causative factor in the late submission of assignments and higher failure rates of online students.

With mobile technologies, it is important for nurse educators to know what is compatible and not compatible for mobile learners. What is viewable on a PC desktop computer may not be viewable when using an iPad® or other tablet device. Providing accessibility to mobile learners is important because more people are using mobile devices to search the Internet, attend class, and read textbooks.

Online Textbook Materials and Software

Knowing and incorporating publisher resources that accompany course textbooks into DE classes can expand the learning possibilities for students. Products that address different learning styles and engage clinical reasoning in students can be found for all levels of educational needs. For graduate and/or doctoral students in nursing, mobile applications supported by websites can be used to improve the educational experience and become essential in clinical practice. Tools ranging from anatomy flashcards to references for laboratory values, patient care algorithms, and certification exam reviews can be used on course websites or handheld technology devices (pdaMD.com, 2010). See Chapter 12 for more information on mobile devices.

SUPPORTING LEARNERS WITH COURSE RESOURCES

Institutions of higher education that seek to develop and retain students in DE programs must consider revising course resources in a manner that centers on the needs of the student and not the system (Ryan, 2001). A systematic review of the enrollment process, addressing details such as payment of fees, communication with staff, departments, and schools, and procurement of learning materials, will detect barriers that deter students from enrolling in, or continuing to attend, DE programs. The idea of a customer relationship management system, mimicking that seen in the business world, could be implemented to support all students, particularly those who live at greater geographic distances (Ryan, 2001). All resources that are available on campus in the live setting should also be available around the clock to DE program students, in a manner that allows the completion of tasks such as academic advising, class registration, and payment of fees. Student-centered resources include e-mail, library access, a bookstore, a faculty and staff directory, and an electronic payment method. Not only does this help students, but providing resources for DE students is also one criterion for accreditation of nursing programs.

E-mail

Upon acceptance to the institution or program, students should receive written communication with contact information for departments and instructors. Generally, in DE programs, the preferred method of course communication is via the institution's student e-mail. However, it is common for students to have multiple e-mail accounts. The institution informs students on the e-mail account used for official school communications. Training or an online tutorial on how to access and use the e-mail system assists students in locating vital communications. Students often use personal e-mail accounts to communicate with faculty. Answering e-mail from student personal e-mail accounts is acceptable, as long as the student is aware that official communications are e-mailed to their student accounts. DE faculty should have some knowledge about the student e-mail system in order to answer minor questions in the online classroom.

Library Access

Many university libraries now have entire collections available in an online format. It is essential for the program's success that DE learners have complete, 24/7 access to collections and databases. When full-text documents are not available in a library's online databases, students will need interlibrary loan services. The library should have a process for providing the loaned materials via e-mail or mailing the items to students' homes. Even when the physical library has print copies, the requested material should be scanned and e-mailed to DE students. Students in DE courses need real-time help from reference librarians to conduct efficient searches, to download materials, and to manage a collection of materials. Many university libraries implement this support by staffing real-time chat inside their virtual libraries. Larger DE programs might want to consider program-specific library personnel designated to handle communication with students.

The use of Google Scholar™ provides DE students access to many scholarly theses, books, abstracts, and articles. For nursing, the Virginia Henderson International Library (nursinglibrary.net/portal/main.aspx) provides abstracts to nursing publications for the general public and access to the actual articles for members of Sigma Theta Tau International. Open Library (openlibrary.org) provides information on over 1 million books. With access to a variety of materials online, the DE learner may need additional instruction for identifying and using scholarly publications.

Bookstore

It is to be expected that students in DE programs may reside at great geographical distances from the campus and be unable to visit college or university bookstores during regular hours of operation. Programs should have systems in place to support DE students, such as the ability to access textbook lists, shop, order, and pay online around the clock. In addition, special rates on shipping of textbooks and other items, such as office supplies and institutional memorabilia, could also be considered for the distance education student.

FACILITATING LEARNER SUCCESS

Student Interaction

Online learning encourages equitable participation of students and allows democratic participation (Gallogly, 2005). However, student interaction requires a course structured to encourage interaction among students and to avoid alienation (Weller, 2002; Swan, Shen, & Hiltz,

2006). Personal connections are established by students for the purposes of emotional support and support during study, and to develop a sense of a shared experience. Research suggests that personal connections among students impact their acquisition experience in the course (Fahy & Ally, 2005) and their motives and intentions. As designers of online courses, nurse educators significantly influence student-to-student interaction. Group and partnered assignments have also been suggested and, when assigned relative to areas of research, may create opportunities for future research partnerships throughout the careers of former students (AACN, 2011).

Faculty Interaction

While peer-to-peer collaboration is important, faculty-to-student interaction remains a key element of successful DE coursework for students. Connection to the instructor is best established at the onset but must be maintained throughout the online course. Course instructors are the initial contact who can reduce anxiety by sharing their own initial fears and experiences related to DE, outlining technical requirements, describing time-management requirements, and making available technical skill training and support personnel (AACN, 2011). Throughout the course, effective DE instructors maintain contact and offer varied communication avenues so that technical difficulties do not delay content questions.

Several aspects of faculty interaction have been highlighted, including a class structure that encourages collaboration and the creation of an online community, promoting collaboration and team problem solving, and establishing a connection to the instructor.

Evaluating Student Support Systems

Billings and Connors (2011) describe the best practices in online learning and recommend a full evaluation of the courses. Most programs have standardized end-of-course evaluations. However, DE programs need additional feedback to evaluate the quality of the DE course. The nurse educator employs this feedback in continued revisions and improvements to the course or program. The six key areas that should be evaluated at the end of each course are access, convenience, connectedness, forming, satisfaction, and proficiency with computer skills.

SUMMARY AND KEY POINTS

Support for the learner in DE programs begins well in advance of enrollment in online coursework. Nursing students of all ages, and particularly nontraditional students who struggle to balance multiple commitments in their pursuit of educational goals, will be satisfied and likely to repeat experiences and recommend institutions with vigorous student support measures built into the DE program. Primary reasons for enrolling in a DE nursing program are flexibility, access, and cost. Primary barriers are technology and technology skills. A solid orientation program can expand students' skills and abilities to do well in the DE classroom. Faculty have a responsibility for planning, implementing, and evaluating DE classes that provide student support systems that enable success.

1. Nursing organizations have called for increasing the number of highly educated RNs, from BSN to the doctoral levels, using technology to do so.
2. It is the role of DE instructors to support students in becoming successful distance learners by providing resources, activities, and courses designed for learner success.
3. Primary reasons for enrolling in a DE program include flexibility in scheduling and geographic location, access to top nursing education, and cost savings.
4. Learner readiness can be assessed using a variety of online quizzes and evaluating the learner's participation in the classroom setting. Readiness to be a successful online learner can be seen in knowledge of course content, adequate participation, and navigation of the classroom and course materials.
5. Enabling factors for students are convenience, flexibility, good time-management skills, and having clearly stated course requirements.
6. Faculty actions that may improve persistence with the class include having a high quality and quantity of interactions with students, showing responsiveness to their needs, and providing clear instructions in all areas of the course.
7. Barriers to online learning include having the equipment and skills needed to attend the DE class and participate. Orienting learners to the DE environment can be done through standardized tutorials and materials or an on-campus meeting (if possible).

8. Providing clear directions and expectations in each course allows the DE student to participate and meet expectations.
9. DE programs must meet Section 508 standards providing the guidelines for software, hardware, Internet, telecommunications, and computers.
10. DE students will attend class 24/7 and need 24/7 technical support. Faculty should be prepared to answer general technical support questions in a timely manner.
11. General resources needed to support the DE learner include e-mail, library access, and methods to pay for courses and books online. Resources should be equivalent to those available to campus-based students.
12. A thorough evaluation of the student experience should be conducted at the end of each course.

REFERENCES

Allen, I., & Seaman, J. (2005). *Growing by degrees—Online education in the United States.* Needham, MA: The Sloan Consortium. Retrieved from http://sloanconsortium.org/resources/growing_by_degrees.pdf

American Association of the Colleges of Nursing (AACN). (2011). *AACN white paper: Technology in nursing education.* Retrieved from http://www.aacn.nche.edu/publications/positions/whitepaper.htm

Atack, L., & Rankin, J. (2002). A descriptive study of registered nurses' experiences with web-based learning. *Journal of Advanced Nursing, 40*(4), 457–465.

Barnard-Brak, L., Lon, W. Y., & Paton, V. (2010). Profiles in self-regulated learning in the online learning environment. *International Review of Research in Open and Distance learning, 11*(1), 61–79.

Billings, D. M. (2000). A framework for assessing outcomes and practices in web-based Courses. *Journal of Nursing Education, 39*(2), 61.

Billings, D. M., & Connors, K. R. (2011). Best practices in online learning. *National League for Nursing Living Book.* Retrieved from http://www.electronicvision.com/nln/chapter02/index.htm

Bouhnik, D., & Marcus, T. (2006). Interaction in distance-learning courses. *Journal of the American Society of Information Science & Technology, 57*(3), 299–305.

Braun, T. (2008). Making a choice: The perceptions and attitudes of online graduate students. *Journal of Technology and Teacher Education, 16*(1), 63–92.

Carruth, A. K., Broussard, P. C., Waldmeier, V. P., Gauthier, D. M., & Mixon, G. (2010). Graduate nursing online orientation course: Transitioning for success. *Journal of Nursing Education, 49*(12), 687–690.

Confessore, G., & Park, L. (2004). Factor validation of the Learner Autonomy Profile (Version 3.0) and extraction of the short form. *International Journal of Self-Directed Learning, 1,* 39–58.

Fahy, P. J., & Ally, M. (2005). Student learning style and asynchronous computer-mediated conferencing (CMC) interaction. *The American Journal of Distance Education, 19*(1), 522.

Frith, K. H., & Kee, C. C. (2003). The effect of communication on nursing student outcomes in a web-based course. *Journal of Nursing Education, 42*(8), 350–358.

Gallogly, J. T. (2005). *Relationship of student satisfaction levels in distance learning and transitional classroom environments at Embry-Riddle aeronautical university*. Unpublished dissertation, University of Central Florida, Orlando, Florida.

Hammond, M. (2005). A review of recent papers on online discussion in teaching and learning in higher education. *Journal of Asynchronous Learning Networks, 9*(3). Retrieved from http://old.sloanconsortium.org/jaln/pdfs/v9n3_hammond.pdf

Holly, C. (2009). The case for distance education in nursing. *MERLOT Journal of Online Learning and Teaching, 5*(3). Retrieved from http://jolt.merlot.org/vol5no3/holly_0909.htm

Jenkins, R. (2011, August 16). Improving online success. *The Chronicle of Higher Education*. Retrieved from http://chronicle.com/blogs/onhiring/improving-online-success/29390?sid=pm&utm_source=pm&utm_medium=en

Marshall, B., & Drummond, M. J. (2006). How teachers engage with assessment for learning: Lessons from the classroom. *Research Papers in Education, 21*(2), 133–149.

McGivny, R. J. (2009). *Adult student persistence in online education: Developing a model to understand the factors that affect student persistence in a course* (Doctoral dissertation). Retrieved from http://scholarworks.umass.edu/cgi/viewcontent.cgi?article=1017&context=open_access_dissertations&sei-redir=1#search=%22persistence%20online%20courses%20definition%22

Moskal, P. D., & Dziuban, C. D. (2001). Present and future directions for assessing cybereducation: The changing research paradigm. In. L. R. Vandervert, L. V. Shavinina, & R. A. Cornell (Eds.), *Cybereducation: The Future of Long-Distance Learning* (pp. 157–184). New York, NY: Mary Ann Liebert.

Parker, A. (2003). Identifying predictors of academic persistence in distance education. *USDLA Journal, 17*(1). 55–62. Retrieved from http://www.usdla.org/html/journal/JAN03_Issue/article06.html

Parkland College. (2011). *Make sure you're ready for an online class*. Retrieved from http://online.parkland.edu/index.cfm?page=ready

Parsad, B., & Lewis, L. (2008). *Distance education at degree-granting postsecondary institutions: 2006–07* (NCES 2009–044). Washington, DC: National Center for Education Statistics, Institute of Education Sciences, U.S. Department of Education. Retrieved from http://nces.ed.gov/pubs2009/2009044.pdf

pdaMD.com. (2010). In the news. Retrieved from http://www.pdamd.com/home

Pennsylvania State University. (2011). *Teaching and learning with technology*. Retrieved from https://esurvey.tlt.psu.edu/Survey.aspx?s=246aa3a5c4b64bb386543eab834f8e75

Rolfe, C. J. (2007). Getting the bugs out of the distance learning experience. *College Quarterly, 10*(3), 1–35.

Ryan, Y. (2001). The provision of learner support services online. In G. M. Farrell (Ed.), *The Changing Faces of Virtual Education* (pp. 71–92). Vancouver, BC: Commonwealth of Learning.

Stanford-Bowers, D. (2008). Persistence in online classes: A study of perceptions among community college stakeholders. *MERLOT Journal of Online Learning and Teaching, 4*(1). Retrieved from http://jolt.merlot.org/vol4no1/stanford-bowers0308.pdf

Sung, K. T. L. (2006). Literature review on self-regulated learning. *Singapore Nursing Journal, 33*(2), 38–45.

Swan, K., Shen, J., & Hiltz, S. R. (2006). Assessment and collaboration in online learning. *Journal of Asynchronous Learning Networks. 10*(1), 45–62. Retrieved from http://sloanconsortium.org/jaln/v10n1/assessment-and-collaboration-online-learning

United States Access Board. (2011). *Electronic and information technology accessibility standards 2000*. Retrieved from http://www.access-board.gov/sec508/standards.htm

University of Houston Distance Education. (2011). TOOLS: Test of Online Learning Success. Retrieved from http://distance.uh.edu/online_learning.html

Watkins, R., Leigh, D., & Triner, D. (2004). Assessing readiness for e-learning. *Performance Improvement Quarterly, 17*(4), 66–79. Retrieved from http://home.gwu.edu/~rwatkins/articles/PIQ2004.pdf

Weller, M. (2002). *Delivering learning on the net. The why, what and how of online education.* London, England, and New York, NY: Routledge Falmer.

WICHE Center for Educational Technology. (2001). *Best practices for electronically offered degree and certificate programs.* Retrieved from http://wcet.wiche.edu/wcet/docs/cigs/studentauthentication/Accrediting_BestPractices.pdf

SIX

Exemplars of Student Support

DEBORAH J. CLARK

Exemplars of student support were developed by sending nurse educators a list of interview questions about their online teaching experiences, particularly experiences with student support. They generously gave of their time and expertise to this chapter. The chapter will present a nurse educator in a DNP and a RN-BSN program.

DNP PROGRAM, UNIVERSITY OF ALABAMA IN HUNTSVILLE: Faye Anderson, DNS, RN, NEA-BC

Dr. Anderson is an associate professor and DNP coordinator at University of Alabama in Huntsville (UAHuntsville). She holds a BS in nursing, a MS in community health nursing, and a DNS with a major in nursing administration. She has 7 years of experience teaching in an associate-degree nursing program and 8 years at UAHuntsville. She started teaching online in 2003 and led the development of an online MSN tract (leadership in health services) and DNP programs; she teaches in both. UAHuntsville currently uses ANGEL® for their learning management system (LMS). Dr. Anderson was neutral about distance education (DE) when she was first assigned to teach an online course. She acknowledges that teaching a course online without prior experience or preparation is less than ideal, but a strong online course can be designed when a faculty member is partnered with an instruction technology specialist. She is now a strong advocate for online education. She continues to enjoy teaching face to face but finds that the same quality of faculty-to-student relationships can be achieved in online courses.

Dr. Anderson's philosophy of teaching has evolved over the years as her experience grew and her own continuing education expanded her knowledge and skills. She believes that a traditional course cannot simply be placed online without making adjustments for the technology and using online teaching strategies. She believes students must be presented with clear content, deadlines, and opportunities for collaboration. If possible, the course should be fully developed before it begins. Changes once a course begins should be rare and quickly communicated to all students. Communication is integral to the online course; student-to-student and student-to-instructor communication in the course are strategies that improve the connection to the course and to faculty. Students should be interacting with each other just as in the traditional classroom setting.

Student Readiness for Online Learning

Although UAHuntsville has no structured process for nursing students to assess their readiness to be online learners before starting the online master's program, there are supports in place for online nursing students. The College of Nursing provides a *Student Handbook for Online Learning* that contains information on resources; technical support telephone numbers; an online tutorial for the LMS; and policies related to communication, academic honesty, and copyright. Within the College of Nursing's *Student Handbook for Online Learning* is a link to the Illinois Online Network's page on "What Makes a Successful Online Student?" (www.ion.uillinois.edu/resources/tutorials/pedagogy/StudentProfile.asp). Students can quickly review whether they match the characteristics of a successful online student. Online nursing students at UAHuntsville attend a required on-campus orientation to their selected program. A portion of this orientation is dedicated to demonstrating the ANGEL platform and accessing the online library. Students can access assistance for using LMS by calling the university's technical support desk; if problems are specific to nursing applications, there is technical support in the College of Nursing.

Enabling Factors for Student Success

When discussing the enabling factors for student success, Dr. Anderson believes that flexibility is the major factor, along with time-management skills and self-discipline. DE programs that are flexible and fit the schedule of a busy working nurse benefit student success. Time-management skills are required to manage multiple assignments across the term, including keeping a calendar and avoiding procrastination. Dr. Anderson has seen students who lack time-management skills be unsuccessful in an online class. Self-discipline is an important requirement, and beginning online students may find this an area for growth. Faculty, through class orientation documents, can provide some guidance to students about how to organize their work for the class and provide examples of how others have been successful by planning their workload for the term.

Surprises do not work well in the distance environment. Students "attend" class at all hours of the day and night and sometimes forget that the instructor is on a different personal schedule. Dr. Anderson believes that instructors do not need to be available 24/7, but instructor availability (all contact information including phone numbers and e-mail) should be posted in the classroom. Dr. Anderson provides clearly stated course requirements, particularly for assignments, participation, and discussion questions. Because there are few, if any, verbal discussions with the DE student, the written directions and instructions must be clear and detailed. In addition, she sees teacher responsiveness in providing timely and thorough grading and feedback of student assignments during that lesson (week or module) as being important. Publishing feedback to students privately, but where they can easily locate the feedback, is a critical element in a DE course.

Dr. Anderson sees computer skills and abilities related to word processing programs, Internet search engines, e-mail, and other applications as foundational to success in a DE program for students and faculty. Although some skills can be learned at orientation or in the first few weeks of class, a lack of skills or access to a reliable computer can negatively influence students' success and their enjoyment of the course. She suggests encouraging students to have a backup computer at a local library, a college campus, or a neighbor's or family member's house. Anderson says, "We have all experienced the occasional 'crash' of a computer—and students will experience this too. A backup computer plan is necessary for distance education nursing students."

Supporting Students to Overcome Barriers to Success

Overall, there is no difference in the student support services between on-campus and DE nursing students. Dr. Anderson describes access to the online library, e-mail, technology help desk, and the College of Nursing support technician. Students also register for their classes online and order their textbooks online. The DNP online students at UAHuntsville have additional access to the libraries of the Alabama University System Libraries because they are enrolled in a joint DNP program. Online learners can also have all interlibrary loan requests e-mailed directly to them. The online learners also can use the university's writing center support staff. Dr. Anderson encourages faculty to know their campus resources for technical support and technology classes. Faculty direct students to these resources once a problem area is identified or a student asks for help.

Dr. Anderson recommends an orientation course for students beginning a DE program, including an overview of the program and specific sessions about the LMS and the online library resources. Providing students with links to other pre-prepared tutorials such as PowerPoint® presentations, netiquette for online communication, and the American Psychological Association (APA) writing style should be made available. Additional classes covering the school e-mail system, online registration, and student account access help students understand the resources at the University.

Dr. Anderson provides strategies to eliminate or prevent social isolation or a sense of alienation in her classes. Students meet each other at the on-campus orientation sessions, and then faculty use a variety of strategies within the courses that promote a sense of community. Students introduce themselves in class and provide some personal and professional background information. Students and faculty can upload a picture of themselves to the online classroom. Dr. Anderson designs group discussions and group assignments that serve to promote the growth of relationships. All of these strategies promote a sense of being in a learning community. As a result of the emphasis on student-to-student interaction, relationships persist even after students complete their programs. One group of DNP students formed a limited liability company (LLC) to provide professional education to others. Other students contact each other to coordinate their attendance at professional meetings. Another group of former DNP students continues to provide peer review of manuscripts and grant proposals.

Adapting to the online classroom is a challenge for nursing students. Acknowledging this challenge, the College of Nursing adopted a standard layout for online courses. Each unit of study follows a format of objectives, learning activities, and assignments. Calendars and schedules in the classroom remind students of due dates and deadlines. Faculty strategies for communicating course materials and information to students include voice-recorded online lectures, live chats with the class, phone conversations, and webcam meetings.

Personal Characteristics That Aid Student Success

Dr. Anderson believes that the quality and quantity of faculty interaction aid student success. She provides faculty-to-student interactions that personalize the course, such as providing a welcome letter with information on her background and experience. She also likes to quickly respond to students and answer their questions. If she is planning to be away from the class, she will give the class prior notice so they will not be waiting for feedback. She posts the course requirements and schedule on the first day of class. When students miss an assignment deadline, she sends them an e-mail request or reminder. Dr. Anderson responds to discussion board assignments as well as provides individualized feedback on assignments. She also uses telephone or face-to-face meetings (for nearby students) to resolve questions or for advisement.

RN-BSN AND MSN PROGRAMS: Crystal Lane-Tillerson, PhD, MEd, MS, RN, CNE

Dr. Crystal Lane-Tillerson is the associate director of ECPI University's online bachelor's degree program for RNs returning to school after receiving their diploma or associate degree in nursing. She is also an adjunct faculty member at Liberty University and Olivet University. In total, she has 6 years of teaching experience, with 5 of those being online. Dr. Lane-Tillerson currently teaches nursing at the undergraduate and graduate levels. In her master's and doctoral studies, she attended two online courses. Her personal interest in DE stems from the exciting opportunity to reach students from all over the country and, in some cases, the world. She is fulfilled as a nurse educator by knowing that she has influenced the practice of many nurses and, ultimately, the care of their patients. Online nursing students additionally benefit because they are able to interact and learn with other students from various demographic locations, work environments, and health care facilities.

Dr. Lane-Tillerson uses Moodle™ and Blackboard™ learning management systems. She is mostly self-taught but continues to learn new functionalities and capabilities on a daily basis. She prepared herself for online teaching by reading articles related to best practices in DE, attending webinars, and taking part in an online social network for online educators. Joining online communities, such as LinkedIn© (specifically in groups for online faculty, university administrators, or instructional designers), provides an opportunity to chat with other online teachers, to share resources and ideas, or just to vent about the online experience. She also prepared by reflecting on the learning conditions of her students, her past personal experience as an online learner, and evidence-based best practices.

Student Readiness for Online Learning

Dr. Lane-Tillerson's personal philosophy about supporting the online learner is based on her experiences in the online environment. She sees effective communication as the single most important element that should always be maintained in the online environment. However, this may also be the most challenging. Clear lines of communication established at the beginning of a course lead to student success. Students expect and deserve timely responses and feedback as needed to foster their success. Online instructors must be available to their students through a variety of means including e-mail, phone, chat, and webcam. Online instructors should communicate regularly with students, on an individual basis and as a group.

Dr. Lane-Tillerson describes one of the challenges in maintaining good communication with students—written communication can be more time consuming than verbal. Lane-Tillerson says, "Standing in front of a classroom of students and telling them everything you wanted them to know takes much less time than guiding students as they discover and develop new knowledge. Questions from students can be addressed quickly, and incidences of miscommunication can be solved with ease in a traditional classroom." However, there are also benefits to written communication. Lane-Tillerson says, "Students who aren't comfortable speaking out in class may be more comfortable asking their question by e-mail, particularly when I reply with specific suggestions."

Dr. Lane-Tillerson also recommends having clear, concise, and meaningful written instructions for the students. Clear expectations and assignment rubrics reduce the number of questions because clear and concise guidance is always available. A grading rubric is a grid that lists the criteria and the possible points to be earned. Rubrics are beneficial for the student and for the faculty grading the assignment. When grading an assignment, instructors place feedback within the assignment as well as the rubric and send both back to the student. Dr. Lane-Tillerson usually sends the graded assignment back within

5 days. Grading rubrics are developed over time, with each use leading to refinement and clarity in instructions. In asynchronous learning environments, where students may need guidance at 3 a.m., providing clear instructions via course documents or grading rubrics may improve the student's overall learning experience and success.

Dr. Lane-Tillerson encourages student engagement. Students need to remain engaged in the educational environment, and studies indicate that this may be more of a challenge in the online environment than in traditional in-seat classrooms (Lorenzo, 2011). Online faculty can use the LMS to track student involvement by assessing their page views in a class. By tracking students on a regular basis, instructors can reach out to students who have not logged into class or who have not posted and let them know that the instructor is there to assist and facilitate learning. Dr. Lane-Tillerson and the other faculty members in the BSN program review their students' class activities on a weekly basis to determine who may need a phone call or other form of communication to keep them engaged and successful.

Enabling Factors for Student Success

To ensure that students understand the requirements of the program, Dr. Lane-Tillerson shared that potential students of the BSN program meet with the director or associate director either in person or by telephone to discuss the requirements of the program before enrolling. A curriculum handout is given to the student, and the discussion includes the challenges of the online environment, the time required to read textbooks and published articles, and the dedication required to be successful in the program. Dr. Lane-Tillerson's BSN students participate in a 2-week, self-paced orientation completed prior to the first day of class. The orientation covers a series of eight mini-lessons on how to access e-mail, use online library services, use the BSN Online Community Group, contact technical support and their faculty, use APA format and avoid plagiarism, communicate in the LMS, and post and respond in the discussion forum. Students submit a check-off form at the end of orientation. Because of the extensive orientation mini-lessons and activities, faculty can verify that students have the necessary computer skills to participate in classes effectively. Lorenzo (2011) described online orientations as an "effective practice that has resulted in better retention rates in community college online programs."

The students are offered as much if not more support than the traditional in-seat students on campus. For example, students have 24-hour access to the online library including the EBSCOhost library database with CINAHL Plus, Health Source: Consumer Edition, Health Source: Nursing Edition, MEDLINE, and the Nursing Reference Center. Students have access to library assistance online via the "Ask the Librarian" feature and the library tutorial. The online library's "How-To" guides and interactive tutorials are available to teach students how to locate, retrieve, and use published research and Internet searching. At the beginning of each term, students hold a videoconference with their instructor to review the course requirements and discuss any questions or concerns they might have. Students are also encouraged to use the webcams for team assignments or to contact their instructors when needed.

Supporting Students to Overcome Barriers to Success

The technical requirements for online BSN students are provided in the online orientation information, college catalog, and BSN student handbook. Once students are enrolled in an online course, the university requires an online survey to measure their readiness to be an online learner and an orientation to LMS. The LMS training provides information regarding how to access the courses, navigate the homepage, participate in class, post to discussion forums, submit an assignment, take an exam, and access the 24/7 technical support.

Flexibility and convenience are important, and Dr. Lane-Tillerson believes that students do find that DE allows for more flexibility of their time. DE is convenient because students can move at their own pace to some extent. Lane-Tillerson says, "It may take one student 30 minutes to view a lecture and take another student 2 hours." Without the constraint of classroom scheduling, students who do not get all of the content information the first time can review it repeatedly until they feel comfortable.

Dr. Lane-Tillerson agrees that students who are good managers of their time are more likely to be successful. In the program's capstone course, Dr. Lane-Tillerson's most valuable advice from past students to future online students is to develop and maintain good time-management skills. Roper (2007) agrees that establishing a dedicated class time helped students to make certain they were devoting enough time for class participation. Roper also noted that self-discipline and limiting distractions aided student success. Dr. Lane-Tillerson encourages her students to set aside time dedicated to class just as if they were sitting in a classroom and to study in a part of their house that has minimal distractions or go to nearby locations to study, such as a public library.

Discussing teacher responsiveness, Dr. Lane-Tillerson suggests that just as instructors require substantial postings from the students, students should expect the same from their instructors. She finds it imperative to provide students with valuable feedback and responses in a timely manner. Students often get discouraged about the DE environment because they feel disconnected from their instructors. Students tend to feel more connected if the instructor posts often and asks questions of individual students based on their posts. This can be helpful if the students are at different levels of understanding or have different learning styles. The instructor can tailor the feedback and questions to the student in question. Dr. Lane-Tillerson emphasizes, "No matter how sophisticated or up-to-date the technology capabilities are, the bottom line is that the instructor still has to teach the student." As suggested by Abel (2005), "it's still the teaching, not the technology" (p. 76. para. 12) that makes a valuable learning experience.

Avoiding social isolation and alienation is accomplished by encouraging students to communicate with the instructor and their classmates via video cameras and open discussion boards. Team assignments in many of the courses require communication among students apart from their regular discussion board communication. Team discussion areas in the course serve as the "meeting room." Dabbagh (2007) suggests, "online learners must be ready to share their work, interact within small and large groups in virtual settings, and collaborate on projects online or otherwise risk isolation in a community growing increasingly dependent on connectivity and interaction" (para. 9).

To support their students, the BSN faculty members are present in their respective course at least 5 days out of the week and post a minimum of three substantive posts that lead the discussion or steer the discussion. Faculty members are also required to "peek" into the class on weekends to see if students have posted any questions or e-mails to them.

E-books are entering DE, and Dr. Lane-Tillerson uses them in some of her classes. Each online course includes resources and contact information available to students who may need assistance with their e-books or other electronic resources. Publishers have their own websites with "help" links that students may access as needed. Being prepared to assist students with basic questions and having technical support available supports learning.

In her discussion regarding considerations made when developing the BSN program, Dr. Lane-Tillerson shared that the content and assignments in most of the BSN courses were designed to build on each other. In this model, as students complete each part of the assignment, they are accomplishing objectives in each unit (week) of the course, which culminates in the course objectives and ultimately the program objectives. For example, in the "Nurse as Educator" course, students, over the course of the term, build a lesson plan using a template. They start in Week 1, selecting a topic and objectives. The assignment culminates in the last week of the course with a full lesson plan that includes objectives, content, resources, teaching materials, and so on. The week's content begins with an overview for the week that includes the required reading, topic outline, objectives, discussion question due dates, and assignment and/or test due dates. In addition to this overview document, the links for each discussion question, assignment and test dates are posted to remind the student of the deadlines.

Personal Characteristics That Aid Student Success

Dr. Lane-Tillerson believes that instructors must be available to their DE students and that students must feel comfortable contacting the instructor when needed. She makes her cell phone number available and provides flexible office hours, which sends the message that the instructor is available for student support when needed. Although not every nurse educator would be comfortable with such access, Dr. Lane-Tillerson says, "It works for me." Interacting with students in synchronous communication activities using virtual chat and videoconferencing encourages students to communicate and reveals that the faculty member is available and supportive (Table 6.1). Table 6.1 provides links to YouTube

TABLE 6.1 YouTube™ Tutorials for Distance Education

Author/Title	URL
CollaborizeClassroom: Tucker, C. How to Engage Students Online, Increase Participation and Improve Discussions	www.youtube.com/watch?v=RzsbSSV4qYk
Fullmer, M. Teaching With Online Discussion Forums	www.youtube.com/watch?v=p3xo1RipS-c
Indiana University. Managing an Online Course: Discussion Forums	www.youtube.com/watch?v=uTpEVLxbcvQ
Rubrics 101: Making Grading a Learning Experience	www.youtube.com/watch?v=_U4rMpUJ8Fo
Towson University: Wizer, D. Designing Engaging Online Events	www.youtube.com/watch?v=gNycUv-LyhY&feature=related

videos, which describe common technology tools to improve student engagement.

Pearls of Wisdom From Our Experts

1. Prepare an orientation course or program prior to the beginning of the first online course
2. Fully develop the course before the first day of class
3. Set up opportunities for student–student and student–instructor communication through class discussions, team projects, web-cam meetings, phone conversations, and e-mail messages
4. Personalize the course with a personal introduction and provide space for students to introduce themselves and share their personal information
5. Provide timely feedback for assignments and questions
6. Know the campus resources and provide links for student use
7. Use prepared tutorials when available on all kinds of topics—writing style, software, libraries, and so on, when available
8. Mix up assignments and class materials to meet all learning style preferences
9. Spend time learning how to facilitate discussions where you acknowledge the learner's post, take advantage of the opportunity to teach something new, apply it to the conversation, and ask critical-thinking or clinical-reasoning questions
10. Clarify and quantify assignments by using well-constructed grading rubrics

REFERENCES

Abel, R. (2005). Implementing best practices in online teaching. *Educause Quarterly, 28*(5), 75–77.

Dabbagh, N. (2007). The online learner: Characteristics and pedagogical implications. *Contemporary Issues in Technology and Teacher education* [Online serial], *7*(3). Retrieved from http://www.citejournal.org/vol7/iss3/general/article1.cfm

Lorenzo, G. (2011). *Online education learner engagement and academic success strategies at community colleges*. Retrieved from http://www.edpath.com/images/OnlineLearning ReportFinal2.pdf

Roper, A. (2007). How students develop online learning skills. *Educause Quarterly, 30*(1), 62–65.

SEVEN

Using Learning Objects to Enhance Distance Education

JEANNE P. SEWELL

The purpose of this chapter is to explore the concept of learning objects including assessing quality, finding and using learning objects when planning online course lessons, and creating learning objects. Finally, there will be a description of searchable database repositories that contain learning objects, lessons, and assignments.

DEFINING LEARNING OBJECTS AND STANDARDS

A learning object is an instructional technology concept that describes a digital item that can be used in a number of different learning contexts by many users at the same time. The term *learning object* was first described by David Wiley (2000) as "any digital resource that can be reused to support learning" (p. 7). Wiley adopted the term *object* from Dahl and Nygaard's (1966) description of a programming language component that can be reused. Learning objects vary in complexity from a small simple animated graphic to a complex digital textbook or an online course.

UNDERSTANDING STANDARDS FOR LEARNING OBJECTS

Learning objects are more complex than printed books or other print learning resources that consist of paper, pictures, diagrams, and printed material. Digital objects require terminology that describes the content of the object (metadata), a format that can be utilized by a computer application (app), a method of retrieval, and a method of storage. For the purpose of this chapter, standards for learning objects will be addressed from the perspective of the data repository, with examples of standards from the Library of Congress, Learning Object Review Instrument (LORI), and the Multimedia Educational Resource for Learning and Online Teaching (MERLOT) peer-review process. The Library of Congress addresses the technical standards for digital resources, whereas LORI and MERLOT address the quality of the digital object standards from the user's perspective as well as the pedagogical perspective.

Library of Congress Standards

According to the Library of Congress, there are four primary standards for digital resources (Library of Congress, n.d.): metadata that describes the content of the item, metadata encoding formats for the item, format to support the long-term preservation of the item, and protocol for search and retrieval of the item. The metadata are the tags, keywords, or descriptors used to find digital resources on the Internet or digital libraries. The metadata is often embedded in the digital resource and invisible to the user. The metadata encoding, in simplistic terms, refers to the type of data, for example, a portable data format (PDF), Movie Picture Expert Group 3 or 4 (MP3 or MP4) digital audio recording file, or a graphic file (.gif). Long-term support of digital resources is challenging but important.

Although there have been no substantial changes in "paper" over the last hundred years, there have been many substantial changes in media over the last 10 years. For example, computers used to have slots for floppy disks. Floppy disks were phased out when CDs (compact disks) became popular. When computer technology advanced to support video, CDs were phased out with the introduction of digital video disks (DVDs) and Blu-ray disks (BDs). The Library of Congress specifies the technical standards for searching and retrieving digital items (memory.loc.gov/ammem/about/techIn.html). Information technology experts have developed applications that comply with standards to make it easy to search for and retrieve digital resources.

LORI Standards

The LORI is a tool used to assess the quality of digital resources in the Canadian Network of Learning Object Repositories (www.elera.net/eLera/Home/About%20%20LORI). eLera is a group of members who use the repositories. Membership is free but requires registration to create a log-in name and password. eLera members use the LORI tool to evaluate the learning objects. The LORI instrument uses a matrix with a rating of five stars, with one star representing low quality and five stars representing the highest quality. The instrument measures nine dimensions of quality, which can be reviewed here: elera.net/eLera/Home/Articles/LORI%201.5.pdf.

MERLOT Peer-Review Standards

MERLOT is an internationally recognized learning object repository found at www.merlot.org/merlot/index.htm. Membership in MERLOT is free but requires registration to create a log-in name and password. Members of MERLOT can use any learning object in its repository. Most of the learning objects have been peer reviewed. The MERLOT peer-review tool uses stars to depict the quality of the learning object, with five stars being best. The MERLOT criteria evaluate the quality of content, potential effectiveness as a teaching–learning tool, and ease of use (taste.merlot.org/evaluationcriteria.html). Each learning object in the MERLOT repository may also include ratings by users (comments), information about the popularity of the learning resource as indicated by the number of member personal collections, and any associated learning exercises.

Creative Commons License

Creative Commons (CC) is a nonprofit organization that provides solutions to allow sharing of digital resources. Prior to the development of CC, open sharing was stifled by the U.S. copyright law, which automatically copyrights just about everything that is stated, written, or created (U.S. Copyright Office, 2008). CC license, on the other hand, supports sharing in order to maximize "... digital creativity, sharing, and innovation" (Creative Commons, n.d., para. 10). The CC licenses address four factors, including acknowledgment of the author, right to modify the work, right to sell the work, and the requirement to use the same license on the new work. There are six types of CC licenses varying from legal open sharing, including allowing modifications with noncommercial and commercial entities with the only stipulation of acknowledging the author, to more restricted sharing acknowledging the author, limited to noncommercial use with absolutely no changes. A description of each of the six licenses can be viewed at creativecommons.org/licenses.

Open Educational Resources

Open educational resources (OERs) refer to online educational materials that are openly licensed for noncommercial use, are of high quality, and can be used and adapted by a community of users (United Nations Educational, Scientific, and Cultural Organization [UNESCO], 2002). The term and definition were agreed upon at the UNESCO meeting in 2002. From the United Nations' standpoint, it was important for individuals who live in remote places and have Internet access to have access to learning resources without any associated financial costs.

The concept of open education developed in the late 1960s and early 1970s, long before the widespread use of computers and the Internet (Hassett & Weisberg, 1972; Tallboy & Shore, 1973). Open education became more popular in higher education, when in Great Britain, the Open University enrolled 24,000 students in 1971 (Howe, 1976). The Open University allowed students in remote places to enroll in college courses, but the learning content was delivered with postal mail, not electronically. It was not until the widespread development of the World Wide Web and the Internet that the concept of digital OERs was developed. The William and Flora Hewlett Foundation is a philanthropic organization that provides grants to support education and the use of OERs. In essence, OERs are learning objects that are free, are of high quality, are sustainable, use a CC share and share-alike license, are of value to developing countries, exist in different media formats, encourage collaboration among users, and are relevant to users (William and Flora Hewlett Foundation, 2011). Types of OERs include open textbooks, open-access research, open journals, open learning resources, and open tools.

Open Textbooks

There are a growing number of open textbooks. According to a study by the Student Public Interest Research Group (PIRG), open textbooks have the potential of reducing the $900 per-year average cost of textbooks by 80% to $184 per year (Allen & Student PIRGS, 2010). There are numerous sources of open textbooks. Many are located in learning object repositories, like MERLOT (www.merlot.org), and others are available from publishers like Flat World Knowledge (www.flatworldknowledge.com). Examples of open textbooks related to the health sciences include *The Whole Brain Atlas* (www.med.harvard.edu/AANLIB/home.html), *Medicines by Design* (publications.nigms.nih.gov/medbydesign), *Nutrition* (docs.google.com/document/d/1uA_tPn4ERObjediVzRkYHLvdomvRyBEAfE0PU4N1Q3Q/edit?hl=en_US#), *ChemWiki* (chemwiki.ucdavis.edu), and *Epidemiology and Prevention of*

Vaccine-Preventable Diseases (www.cdc.gov/vaccines/pubs/pinkbook/default.htm#download). Open textbooks are available in a number of formats, such as websites, PDF files, Google Docs, and wikis.

There are pluses and minuses associated with open textbooks. In addition to saving costs, open textbooks can be used as a component of a learning activity. For example, students could add to a textbook on disaster management with current events involving disaster management after the hurricanes that tore through Alabama, Georgia, and Joplin, Missouri, and the floods that ravaged North Dakota during 2011. Websites such as Writing Spaces (writingspaces.org) allow instructors and students to create open textbooks with peer-reviewed collections of essays on writing. Open textbooks have drawbacks when used for education. Instructors have to review the books to ensure the accuracy and reliability of the information. Open textbooks have not necessarily gone through the editing and peer-review processes of the commercial publisher (Baker & Hood, 2011).

Open-Access Research

Open-access research is an emerging concept for redistributing scholarship. In 2008, the National Institutes of Health (NIH) accepted a policy that requires recipients of NIH funding to submit final peer-review manuscripts accepted for publication to PubMed Central (U.S. Department of Health and Human Services, n.d.). Research findings are also available from the National Science Foundation (www.nsf.gov/index.jsp).

Open Journals

Open journals are another emerging concept for redistributing scholarship using the Internet. Repositories with searchable links to open-access journals include Directory of Open Access Journals (DOAJ; www.doaj.org), BioMed Central (www.biomedcentral.com), Oxford Journals (www.oxfordjournals.org/oxfordopen), Public Knowledge Project (PKP; pkp.sfu.ca), and Bentham Open (www.benthamscience.com/open). The DOAJ repository has a listing of open-access journals pertinent to nursing written in many of the world languages. Examples of some popular open journals pertinent to nursing and online teaching are noted in Table 7.1.

TABLE 7.1 Online Journals Pertinent to Nursing and Online Learning

Journal	Website
Online Journal of Issues in Nursing	nursingworld.org/OJIN
Online Journal of Nursing Informatics	www.ojni.org
Journal of Online Learning and Teaching	jolt.merlot.org

Open Learning

Open learning refers to free online courses and other digital lessons that are available to anyone who wants to access them. Open learning resources range from entire online courses, such as the OpenCourseWare project, to online lessons available through iTunes and iTunes U.

OpenCourseWare

The Massachusetts Institute of Technology (MIT) shocked the higher education community when it announced the open distribution of its university-level courses on the Internet in 2001 (MIT OpenCourseWare, 2011). In 2008, the OpenCourseWare Consortium was formed as an independent nonprofit organization (OpenCourseWare Consortium, n.d.). Today, the consortium represents over 250 universities worldwide and has published over 13,000 courses in 20 different languages. The stated aspiration for the OpenCourseWare Consortium is to create "the tools to bridge the global gap between human potential and opportunity, so that motivated people everywhere can improve their lives and change the world" (OpenCourseWare Consortium, 2011, para. 12).

iTunes and iTunes U

iTunes®, created by Apple®, is an app that allows users to sync music, audio files, e-books (electronic books), movies, PDF files, and more between a laptop or desktop computer and a portable media device, such as a tablet or smartphone. The iTunes app can be used with the Mac and Windows operating systems. There are many free learning resources available from the iTunes store. New iTunes users should consider reviewing the many video tutorials online at www.apple.com/itunes/how-to.

iTunes U is a resource available from the iTunes store. As of 2011, more than 800 universities were openly distributing learning materials in iTunes U. In addition to university learning resources, iTunes includes learning materials from museums, such as the Museum of Modern Art (MoMA), public broadcasting service (PBS) stations, and libraries, such as the New York Public Library (Apple, 2011). To discover open learning resources for nursing in iTunes and iTunes U, use the search feature located in the iTunes store.

Open Tools

Open tools refer to apps that can be used to create and to display the learning content. Apps that can be used to create learning content (learning objects) and available at no charge are discussed later in this chapter.

There are many open app tools available to display learning content, for example, learning management systems (LMSs). Examples of open tools are Moodle™ (moodle.org), Sakai (sakaiproject.org), OLAT (www.olat.org), Canvas (www.instructure.com), and ATutor® (atutor.ca).

MATCHING LEARNING OBJECTS TO LESSON OUTCOMES

In order to optimize learning, it is very important to match learning objects to lesson outcomes. Educators commonly use Bloom's Taxonomy of Learning or the revision by Anderson and Krathwohl to identify learning outcomes. Bloom conceptualized learning occurring at six levels—knowledge, comprehension, application, analysis, synthesis, and evaluation (Bloom, 1956). Bloom identified that higher-order thinking skills were used at the analysis, synthesis, and evaluation levels, with evaluation being the highest order. Anderson and Krathwohl revised Bloom's taxonomy and used slightly different wording (Anderson, Krathwohl, & Bloom, 2001). They identified higher-order thinking skills as analyzing, evaluating, and creating, with creating being the highest. Chapter 10 contains more information.

How people learn is another aspect to consider when matching learning objects to learning outcomes. People have learning preferences. Dale's Cone of Experience provides a mental model about how people learn (see Figure 7.1). Dale's Cone of Experience is based upon the 1946 work of Edgar Dale (Thalheimer, 2006). The original model did not include any numbers. It is not evidence based, and while popular, its use to explain learning is very controversial. In actuality, people's learning preferences are very individual (Sewell & Thede, 2013). It is important to understand that higher-order thinking skills are based upon knowledge and comprehension. Individuals practice learning in order to retain it and apply it to new situations. Students at the undergraduate and graduate levels who are taking courses with new terminology and new concepts may benefit from learning objects that are directed at lower-order thinking skills.

Knowledge/Remembering

Quizzes are useful in assisting learners to know and remember. Quiz questions focus on definitions or identification of terms used to describe parts of a graphic. There are several interactive online tools that allow users to create and share flashcards with others. Examples of online

FIGURE 7.1 Dale's Cone of Experience. Reprinted with permission from Pastore (2003).

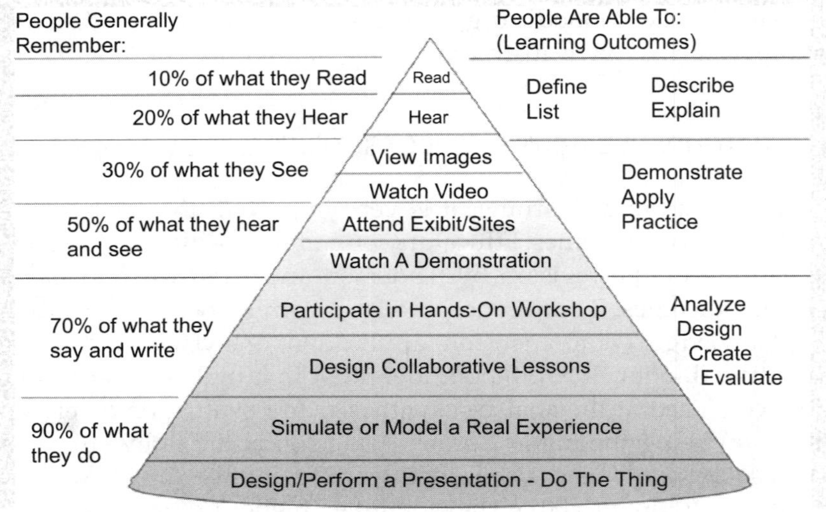

People Generally Remember:		People Are Able To: (Learning Outcomes)
10% of what they Read	Read	Define, List, Describe, Explain
20% of what they Hear	Hear	
30% of what they See	View Images; Watch Video	Demonstrate, Apply, Practice
50% of what they hear and see	Attend Exibit/Sites; Watch A Demonstration	
70% of what they say and write	Participate in Hands-On Workshop; Design Collaborative Lessons	Analyze, Design, Create, Evaluate
90% of what they do	Simulate or Model a Real Experience; Design/Perform a Presentation - Do The Thing	

resources include Quizlet™ (quizlet.com), Flashcard Machine (www.flashcardmachine.com), and Flashcard Exchange (www.flashcardexchange.com). Mouse Party, a Flash game (learn.genetics.utah.edu/content/addiction/drugs/mouse.html), allows users to have a basic understanding about how drug abuse affects the brain.

Comprehension/Understanding

Simulations, animations, and tutorials are helpful to assist learners to achieve outcomes at the comprehension level. Outbreak at Water's Edge: A Public Health Simulation Game (www.mclph.umn.edu/watersedge) is an interactive game and simulation that allows the player to try to discover the source of water contamination making people sick. The materials on hemodialysis at www.kidneypatientguide.org.uk/site/HDanim.php and peritoneal dialysis at www.kidneypatientguide.org.uk/site/pdanim.php are animations. Although the target audience is people with kidney disease, the animations would be very helpful as an introduction for nursing students. ECG (electrocardiogram) at nobelprize.org/educational/medicine/ecg is a simulation game that allows the user to place leads on a patient having a 12-lead ECG and perform simplistic interpretations.

Application/Applying

Interactive tutorials, simulations, instructional games, and case studies can be effective learning methods to assist the learner in applying knowledge. The MedCalc tutorial at www.m2hnursing.com/MedCal/module1_2.php is a tutorial designed to assist nursing students to learn how to calculate medications ranging from simple math to conversions and intravenous flow rates. Construction of the Cell Membrane at www.wisc-online.com/objects/ViewObject.aspx?ID=AP1101 allows the learner to construct a cell with the correct molecules. University of Minnesota hosts a site, Web Anatomy, at msjensen.cehd.umn.edu/WEBANATOMY, with many games that allow learners to apply knowledge on human anatomy. The ABG Tutorial at www.m2hnursing.com/ABG/basic_questions.php provides learners with multiple case studies and enables them to apply knowledge about acid–base balances associated with arterial blood gases.

Higher-Order Thinking Skills

Higher-order thinking skills allow learners to analyze and evaluate the learning content in order to construct new meaning. Learning objects such as multiple-choice questions, computer simulations, and virtual labs designed to assess critical thinking can be effective learning tools. Rice Virtual Lab in Statistics simulations at onlinestatbook.com/rvls.html could be used to allow students to analyze statistical data. DataFerrett (Federated Electronic Research Review, Extraction, and Tabulation Tool) at dataferrett.census.gov could be used to assist students with data analysis. The Chemistry Collective at www.chemcollective.org includes virtual labs and learning activities that could be used to address higher-order thinking skills.

FINDING PUBLISHER AND INTERNET LEARNING OBJECTS

Most nursing and health care textbook publishers include access to online learning objects. The types of objects vary widely compared to online courses that use the associated textbook, for example, full-text journal articles to supplement textbook chapter content, graphics used in the textbook, digital slide shows for chapter content, test-bank questions with rationales and answers, and interactive games. Some textbook publishers provide course files that can be imported by popular LMSs.

Many of the print nursing textbooks and reference books are accompanied with a CD or DVD with learning resources or include information in the book about how to access the publisher's website with student digital learning resources. E-books may also be accompanied by learning resources. One way to for instructors to discover learning objects from publishers is to obtain a log-in name and password to access the publisher's faculty website. Usually, the request has to be approved by the area representative and may take from a few hours to a couple of days. The request process is necessary to ensure security of instructor resources.

MINING THE INTERNET FOR APPROPRIATE LEARNING OBJECTS

There are many learning object databases freely available for users. In 1997, the California State University for Distributed Learning developed MERLOT, a shared-access database for free learning objects. In 2000 MERLOT established discipline-specific editorial boards to conduct peer reviews of the learning objects. Initiatives to support the repository have spawned international use, global partners, and affiliates. To enable searches of other databases with educational resources, MERLOT includes a federated search function. The term *federated search* refers to the ability to search multiple databases simultaneously. As of August, 2012, users could search 13 other learning object collections including Flickr®, YouTube™, and MIT OpenCourseWare; 3 GLOBE (Global Learning Objects Brokered Exchange) partner databases located in Europe, Canada, and Japan; 2 physics databases; 2 faculty development databases; and 2 information technology databases (MERLOT, 2012). Table 7.2 lists other selected learning object repositories and the associated URLs.

PLANNING, CREATION, STORAGE, AND RETRIEVAL OF LEARNING OBJECTS

As noted earlier, the expected learning outcomes should drive the need to use a learning object. In some cases, the instructor may prefer to create a learning object. There are numerous software applications, some free, available to facilitate the creation of new learning objects. Creating new learning objects entails consideration for how the resource will be shared, where objects will be stored, and how they will be retrieved.

When planning a new learning object, it is best for the designer to be familiar with learning objects that have already been created and

TABLE 7.2 Examples of Learning Object Repositories

Name of Repository	Website Address
Connexions—Rice University	cnx.org
EducaNext	www.educanext.org
FREE—Federal Resources for Educational Excellence	www.free.ed.gov
Harvey Project	opencourse.org/Collaboratories/harveyproject
Ide@s	www.ideas.wisconsin.edu/index.cfm
iTunes U	www.apple.com/education/itunes-u
Library of Congress	www.loc.gov/library/libarch-digital.html
MERLOT	www.merlot.org
MIT OpenCourseWare	ocw.mit.edu/index.htm
MLX—Maricopa Learning Exchange	www.mcli.dist.maricopa.edu/mlx
NEAT—Nursing Education and Technology Project	webcls.utmb.edu/neat
Nursing Objects Library—Maricopa Community Colleges Nursing Program	www.mesacc.edu/dept/d31/nursing/learning_objects
Problem-based learning at University of Delaware	primus.nss.udel.edu/Pbl
PBS Teachers	www.pbs.org/teachers
Free e-books by Project Gutenberg	www.gutenberg.org/wiki/Main_Page
Shareable learning objects from WSU College of Nursing and Health	www.wright.edu/nursing/shareableobjects
SMETE	www.smete.org/smete
SoftChalk Connect	www.softchalkconnect.com
Learning Tools	www.learningtools.arts.ubc.ca
The Orange Grove: Florida's K20 Digital Repository	www.theorangegrove.org/index.asp
USG Share	usgshare.org/logon.do
Virginia Commonwealth University School of Nursing learning objects	www.nursing.vcu.edu/it/learning_objects.html
Wisc-Online	www.wisc-online.com

shared. Novice designers should keep the initial design simple—both for the instructor and the student. A good way to begin is to emulate a similar type of learning object already established with the expected learning outcomes in mind. A well-designed learning object includes a stated purpose, learning outcomes, and a list of any special hardware or software requirements. For example, designing a set of flashcards might take 15 minutes, but designing an interactive tutorial with audio and video might take several days or several months.

Creation of new learning objects is easiest with software applications dedicated to that purpose. When creating learning objects, it is often important to show the learner with screenshots, video, or audio clips. There are several powerful apps that are available for download with no charge; Jing®, Audacity®, Hot Potatoes™, and Quandary™ are examples. The MERLOT Content Builder website is also available to users without any fees. Office suite software, Apple iWork® and Microsoft® Office, often used on computers with Mac and Windows operating systems, can also be used to create learning objects. Examples of learning objects with Office software include slide shows with interactive learning activities. The slide show might include an unfolding case study with questions that branch to pertinent information based upon the learner's response. Spreadsheet software could be used to create medication calculation learning activities. Word-processing and slide-show software could be used to create tutorials with graphics and sound.

Jing to Capture Screenshots and Share With Others

Jing (www.techsmith.com/jing/free) allows users to do screen captures of a window or a section on a web page. Jing is available for both Windows and Mac operating systems. Users can "draw" and include text on the screen captures and then share the results with others as an embedded code on sites like Screencast.com® (screencast.com) and Flickr (www.flickr.com). Screencast.com is a cloud computing server that provides users with 2 GB of storage space without a fee, and Flickr is a photo-sharing website.

Audacity to Record and Edit Audio

Audacity (audacity.sourceforge.net) is a free audio recorder and editor available for Windows and Mac operating systems. The app includes tutorials to shorten the learning curve; however, its use is intuitive for many. Audacity can be used to create audio podcasts, which the learner can download from the LMS into most popular media players. Audio podcasts can provide students with a method for learning while commuting to work or exercising.

Hot Potatoes and Quandary to Create Interactive Learning Objects

There is software available specifically for use in creating interactive learning resources. Hot Potatoes (hotpot.uvic.ca) allows users to create learning objects, such as interactive short-answer and multiple-choice questions, crossword puzzles, matching/ordering, and gap-fill exercises. The Hot Potatoes app is freeware and is available for Windows and Mac operating systems. Quandary is freeware that allows users to create action-based mazes that facilitate problem solving. Tutorials and examples for Quandary are online at www.halfbakedsoftware.com/quandary_tutorials_examples.php.

MERLOT Content Builder to Create Learning Objects

MERLOT now includes a Content Builder, which allows designers to create and store personally designed learning objects on a MERLOT server. The Content Builder works with both Windows and Mac operating systems. Help files and tutorials are available at taste.merlot.org/Programs_and_Projects/ContentBuilder.html. Since the learning object is created and stored on a MERLOT server, the creator does not need to worry about finding server space to host the file. This makes creating web pages and associated learning objects easy and convenient for nursing instructors.

Apple iWork to Create E-books and Podcasts

There are several apps on Mac computers that are very useful for creating learning objects. Creating an e-book learning object with an ePub file extension that can be read by e-book reader apps is easy with Apple Pages®, the word processor included with the iWork office suite. Users simply select "ePub" from the "File Export" menu. Saving a file as an ePub works only on the laptop or desktop app but not on Pages for mobile devices.

Likewise, users can use Keynote®, the presentation software included with iWork, to create podcasts with video and audio. A podcast can be created using a Keynote slide show with recorded audio. The completed slide show and recording are sent to iTunes as a podcast. If it is important to customize and edit the audio, the slide show and recording can be sent to GarageBand®, a robust app that can be used for audio recording and editing. GarageBand is not a part of the iWork suite. The "Help" menus in Keynote and GarageBand and the Apple website tutorials assist users to be successful. Keynote and GarageBand are also available for mobile devices, for example, the iPad®, iPod® touch, and iPhone®. Since iTunes is available for Macs and PCs, users with any mobile device can view and listen to podcasts created with Keynote and GarageBand.

Microsoft Office to Create Slide Shows With Audio and Video

Microsoft Office software for the Windows operating system is not as robust as iWork on the Mac. Microsoft users need to search for alternative software in order to create ePub files, such as Lexcycle (www.lexcycle.com/faq/how_to_create_epub). However, users can create slide shows with audio and video using Microsoft Office PowerPoint®. A new feature of PowerPoint version 2010 also allows users to edit the video. There are several Internet tutorials to assist users, for example, office.microsoft.com/en-us/videos/video-create-and-edit-shapes-in-powerpoint-VA101956376.aspx and www.addictivetips.com/windows-tips/powerpoint-2010-tutorial-video-editing.

Commercial Apps for Creating Interactive Learning Objects

There are several commercial apps to create interactive learning objects. Two examples are StudyMate Author® and SoftChalk™. StudyMate Author is designed specifically for creating interactive learning activities. SoftChalk is designed to create online lessons that include the creation of interactive learning activities.

StudyMate Author, a Respondus® product, allows users to create 10 types of interactive Flash® learning activities and games with a couple of clicks of a mouse (Respondus, 2011). Flash is an animation tool. Sample learning activities are available at www.respondus.com/studymate/samples.shtml. The learning activities are based on content with terms and the associated definitions and/or multiple-choice-type questions. The learning content can be keyed into StudyMate Author or imported from files using word-processing or other question-database file formats. Creators can incorporate the use of graphics and audio within the learning activities. Instructors can "publish" the learning activities and games directly into most LMSs, such as Blackboard and Angel. Video tutorials are available at www.respondus.com/products/demos-sm.shtml.

SoftChalk is a comprehensive e-learning authoring system (SoftChalk LLC, 2011a). Like StudyMate Author, the app is easy to learn and use. Users can create professional magazine-like lessons that include coordinated font color and size, paragraph heading styles, and a navigation system. The learning content can be added to the lesson from a word-processing document or keyed into the app window. SoftChalk features allow the creator to include "mouse-over" explanations of terminology using text, hyperlinks, and/or graphics. SoftChalk allows users to create 17 different interactive learning objects and 6 types of quiz questions within the lesson design (SoftChalk LLC, 2011b). Using a federated search tool, creators can import other learning resources from numerous repositories such as YouTube, Flickr, and MERLOT into lessons. The completed lessons can be imported into the file manager of most LMSs or saved to a CD or DVD.

Sharable Content Object Reference Model

The Sharable Content Object Reference Model (SCORM) refers to a set of technical standards that allows authored learning content to work with any LMS. SCORM, developed by the Advanced Distributed Learning for the Department of Defense in 2004, has four functional requirements: interoperability, accessibility, durability, and reusability (Advanced Distributed Learning, n.d.). Hot Potatoes, Quandary, StudyMate Author, and SoftChalk are all SCORM compliant. When a learning object is packaged in the SCORM format, it is saved as a .zip (compressed) file. The SCORM package that is imported into the LMS will be visible from "SCORM" on the course menu. Results from learning activities that are graded or scored can be viewed in the LMS grade book as a separate tab. In essence, SCORM packages allow the instructor and students to receive feedback in the course grade book about interactive learning activities.

SUMMARY AND KEY POINTS

This chapter covered the concept of learning objects in a variety of different directions. Learning objects are synonymous with digital learning resources and learning materials. Nurse educators should take the time to review available learning objects, invest time in developing targeted learning objects for specific courses, and share the learning objectives in one or more available repositories. Since the spirit of creating and using learning objects is sharing, users and creators should contribute the learning objects to repositories.

Key Points

1. To address quality, learning object data repository leadership has developed standards.
2. CC is a nonprofit organization developed to have a legal means to circumvent the U.S. copyright law so that learning objects could be shared by users.
3. OERs are a category of learning objects that include open textbooks, open-access research, open journals, open learning resources, and open tools.
4. In order for learning objects to be effective, the instructor must match the type of learning object to the lesson outcomes. Bloom's taxonomy and the revised taxonomy by Anderson and Krathwohl are used to plan learning outcomes.
5. Learning objects can be discovered from textbook publishers, the Internet, and learning object repositories.

REFERENCES

Advanced Distributed Learning. (n.d.). *Frequently asked questions about SCORM*. Retrieved July 4, 2011, from http://www.adlnet.gov/Documents/SCORM%20FAQ.aspx#scormq1

Allen, N., & Student PIRGS. (2010). *A-cover-to-cover-solution: How open textbooks are the path to textbook affordability*. Retrieved July 1, 2011, from http://www.studentpirgs.org/uploads/66/4d/664d09ba9bc97cc9138eda5faac5e061/A-Cover-To-Cover-Solution.pdf

Anderson, L. W., Krathwohl, D. R., & Bloom, B. S. (2001). *A taxonomy for learning, teaching, and assessing: A revision of Bloom's taxonomy of educational objectives* (Complete ed.). New York: Longman.

Apple. (2011). *iTunes U—A weath of knowledge from top institutions*. Retrieved July 2, 2011, from http://www.apple.com/education/itunes-u/whats-on.html

Baker, J., & Hood, J. (2011, March 8). 7 things you should know about open textbook publishing. *EDUCAUSE*. Retrieved from http://www.educause.edu/Resources/7ThingsYouShouldKnowAboutOpenT/225383

Bloom, B. S. (1956). *Taxonomy of educational objectives: The classification of educational goals* (1st ed.). New York, NY: Longmans, Green.

Creative Commons. (n.d.). Creative Commons. Retrieved June 25, 2011, from http://creativecommons.org/

Dahl, O. J., & Nygaard, K. (1966). SIMULA: An ALGOL-based simulation language. *Communications of the ACM, 9*(9), 671–678. Retrieved from http://cs-exhibitions.uni-klu.ac.at/fileadmin/template/documents/text/simula_an_algol_based_simulation_language.pdf

Hassett, J. D., & Weisberg, A. (1972). *Open education; Alternatives within our tradition.* Englewood Cliffs, NJ: Prentice-Hall.

Howe, H. (1976). Openess—The new kick in education. In G. Thibadeau (Ed.), *Opening up education: A theoretical and practical guide to the open classroom* (p. 7). Dubuque, IA: Kendall/Hunt Pub. Co.

Library of Congress. (n.d.). *Digital library standards.* Retrieved June 29, 2011, from http://www.loc.gov/library/digitalstandards.html

MERLOT. (2012). Search other libraries. Retrieved August 15, 2012, from http://fedsearch.merlot.org/fedsearch/fedsearch.jsp

MIT OpenCourseWare. (2011). *Free online course materials: A decade of open sharing.* Retrieved April 28, 2011, from http://ocw.mit.edu/about/next-decade/

OpenCourseWare Consortium. (2011, March). *The OCW Consortium newsletter.* Retrieved May 15, 2011, from http://ocw.mit.edu/about/newsletter/archive/2011-03/

OpenCourseWare Consortium. (n.d.). *About the OpenCourseWare Consortium.* Retrieved July 2, 2011, from http://ocw.mit.edu/about/ocw-consortium/

Pastore, R. S. (2003). *Principles of teaching.* Retrieved July 8, 2011, from http://teacherworld.com/potdale.html

Respondus. (2011). *StudyMate Author 2.0.* Retrieved July 3, 2011, from http://www.respondus.com/products/studymate.shtml

Sewell, J.P. & Thede, L.Q. (2013). Informatics and nursing: Opportunities and challenges (4th ed.). Philadelphia, PA: Wolters Kluwer.

SoftChalk LLC. (2011a). *SoftChalk.* Retrieved July 3, 2011, from http://softchalk.com/

SoftChalk LLC. (2011b). *SoftChalk features.* Retrieved July 3, 2011, from http://softchalk.com/features

Tallboy, F., & Shore, B. M. (1973). *Open education: Review of the literature and selected annotated bibliography.* Montreal, Canada: McGill University.

Thalheimer, W. (2006, May 1). *People remember 10%, 20%...Oh really?* Retrieved July 8, 2011, from http://www.willatworklearning.com/2006/05/people_remember.html

U.S. Copyright Office. (2008). *Copyright basics.* Retrieved July 1, 2011, from http://www.copyright.gov/circs/circ1.pdf

U.S. Department of Health and Human Services. (n.d.). *National Institutes of Health Public Access.* Retrieved July 1, 2011, from http://publicaccess.nih.gov/

UNESCO. (2002, July). Retrieved March 5, 2011, from http://unesdoc.unesco.org/images/0012/001285/128515e.pdf

Wiley, D. A. (2000). Connecting learning objects to instructional design theory: A definition, a metaphor, and a taxonomy. *Learning Technology, 2830*(435), 1–35. Retrieved from http://www.mendeley.com/research/connecting-learning-objects-to-instructional-design-theory-a-definition-a-metaphor-and-a-taxonomy/

William and Flora Hewlett Foundation. (2011). *Open educational resources.* Retrieved July 3, 2011, from http://www.hewlett.org/programs/education-program/open-educational-resources

EIGHT

Using Simulations to Enhance Clinical Reasoning and Judgment

PAMELA R. JEFFRIES, DIANE S. ASCHENBRENNER, KRISTINA THOMAS DREIFUERST, DESIREE HENSEL, CHRIS KEENAN, and JOYCE B. VAZZANO

Nurses possessing clinical reasoning and judgment have a positive impact on patient outcomes; conversely, nurses lacking clinical reasoning and judgment may not detect acute patient changes and complications, resulting in patient harm and poor-quality care (Aiken, Clarke, Cheung, Sloane, & Silber, 2003). Facilitating the development of clinical reasoning skills is a critical responsibility of nurse educators. In the literature, clinical reasoning is used interchangeably with clinical judgment, problem solving, decision making, and critical thinking (Tanner, 2006; Dowding & Thompson, 2003). A commonality of these definitions is the idea that the nurse has the responsibility to collect cues, process information, come to an understanding of a patient problem or situation, plan and implement interventions, and reflect on this process (Levett-Jones, 2010; Tanner, Padrick, Westfall, & Putzier, 1987).

Opportunities to develop and apply clinical reasoning skills have historically been limited to a real-world setting. Providing students with opportunities to develop clinical reasoning in clinical settings can be challenging because of the unpredictable nature of the health care environments, the safety factors and liability concerns in caring for real human patients, and competing demands for clinical sites (Rhodes & Curran, 2005). These challenges impact the opportunity for students to learn clinical reasoning skills; therefore, new approaches need to be developed. Experiential learning, through the use of clinical simulations and distance education, are options available in contemporary teaching approaches to develop clinical reasoning in students. This chapter will provide information on clinical teaching using distance learning and emerging technologies, such as the use of clinical simulations for developing nursing students' clinical reasoning skills.

OVERVIEW OF CLINICAL REASONING AND CLINICAL JUDGMENT

Mastery of clinical reasoning and clinical judgment is a milestone of professional development as the student nurse moves toward becoming a novice clinician and eventually an expert practitioner. Clinical reasoning and judgment are complex concepts. Clinical reasoning involves reflective thinking and decision-making processes within a clinical situation that informs judgment, action, and response (Facione & Facione, 2008; Tanner, 2006). Knowledge, cognitive skills, reflective inquiry, and metacognition all comprise clinical reasoning (Higgs & Jones, 2008). Clinical reasoning is also the ability to gather and comprehend data while recalling knowledge, skills, and attitudes about a situation as it unfolds (INASCL Board of Directors, 2011). Development of clinical reasoning and judgment in distance learners can be supported through the use of various types of simulation and debriefing experiences.

Clinical judgment is contextual decision making (INASCL Board of Directors, 2011). It is an interpretation of the assessment of the clinical situation and associated action or response (Tanner, 2006). Clinical judgments are "those thinking and evaluative processes that focus on a nurse's response to a patient's ill-structured and multilayered problems" (Lasater, 2007, p. 269). Tanner's (2006) model of clinical judgment includes noticing, interpreting, responding, and reflecting as core concepts. The terms clinical reasoning and clinical judgment are often used interchangeably in the literature; however, they are not identical but, rather, reciprocal. Clinical reasoning informs judgment, clinical judgment informs reasoning, and critical thinking is foundational to both. Critical thinking, as defined by the American Association of Colleges of Nursing (1998) is a process that includes all or part of analysis, synthesis, interpretation, inference, inductive and deductive reasoning, intuition, application, and creativity.

Simulation provides an active learning environment for students to experience clinical situations and to make use of cognitive, affective, and psychomotor skills and, at the same time, practice critical thinking, clinical decision making, and clinical judgment in the context of the (virtual) patient care environment without risk to actual patients (Childs & Sepples, 2006; Jeffries, 2008; Larew, Lessans, Spunt, Foster, & Covington, 2006). It is this interactive learning environment that can be used to develop clinical reasoning and judgment in students, because the simulated patient responds to the student, and it is a safe learning environment. The student can repeat the experience, changing responses and outcomes without creating danger to real human patients. Students learn the patterns, responses, and clinical outcomes associated with those decisions (Childs & Sepples, 2006; Larew et al., 2006).

Clinical reasoning includes higher thinking skills and metacognitive elements. Metacognition, or thinking about thinking in a deep and meaningful way, is a complex process of reflection on the cognitive experiences involved in learning. It can be an active or tacit activity. Thought processes are the cornerstone of reasoning. Clinical reasoning is logical thinking within a clinical context in ways that make them meaningful. This thinking ranges from inductive and deductive strategies to the complex process of analysis, inference, and evaluation (Facione & Facione, 2008).

Clinical reasoning also involves reflective and cognitive process where the clinician uses prior knowledge and assessment and analysis of the client to make an informed response. Reflection based on experience and prior knowledge provides the criteria for knowing the variance from the expected in any given experience (Kane, Sandretto, & Heath, 2004). It can be reflection in action occurring concurrently in the clinical setting and reflection on action that happens after the event when reviewing and recalling activities and decision making (Schön, 1983). Finally it can be reflection beyond action, where anticipation of variance and experience are considered prior to a new experience but based on what has already happened (Dreifuerst, 2009). Critical reflection is attained when students and practitioners question underlying assumptions and understandings, and there is a transformation of meaning that leads to action (Decker, 2007). Distance learners can be guided through the processes of thinking in action, thinking on action, and thinking beyond action through the use of unfolding cases, debriefing, and guided reflection activities.

Demonstration of clinical reasoning can involve framing, heuristic processing, intuition, and clinical grasp. Framing is the thinking activity of organizing and manipulating recognizable categories with the information the brain is receiving. It involves building mental models that enable the learner to further analyze and interpret the elements of a clinical situation, which enhances learning and facilitates generalization to future situations (Teekman, 2000). Framing informs action because it provides contextual meaning to options for addressing the clinical situation at hand. This is evident not only in familiar circumstances but also in unfamiliar ones.

Heuristic processing is a form of experiential problem solving (Klein, 1999). The use of patterns of thinking and a corresponding stacking of activities have been identified as strategies that nurses use to cope with the complexity of patient care environments (Ebright, Patterson, Chalko, & Render, 2003). One such pattern, forward thinking, is an example of the anticipatory nature of clinical reasoning that also relies on the nurse's judgment to inform decision making in clinical situations. Students in distance learning environments can practice stacking strategies and forward-thinking techniques using complex case studies in tandem with simulations independently and through group activities.

Intuition, a hallmark of the expert nurse, is application of knowledge without active cognition of the process of doing so (Dreyfus & Dreyfus, 1986). The expert nurse demonstrates intuition through rapid, tacit recognition of the salient aspects of a clinical situation with subsequent informed decision making (Benner, 1984). It is as if they do not have to think about it; they just have a sense of knowing what is occurring and how to respond. This is similar to the concept of the clinical grasp where, through experience, the nurse learns to chunk or combine salient pattern recognition and trigger an established response through developing knowledge and repeated exposure (Ebright et al., 2003). Nonetheless, expertise is a product of experience, and knowing is reflection and anticipation demonstrated through clinical reasoning. Experiential learning opportunities for distance students that teach pattern recognition and unfolding case information can foster this expertise and build foundational knowledge from which the clinical reasoning and judgment can develop.

In this way, clinical reasoning informs decision making, which is the essence of judgment. Clinical judgments are thinking and evaluative processes based on the response of the nurse to the assessment of the patient and the situation (Lasater, 2007). Through judgment, the nurse recognizes salient clinical data and develops a clinical decision, an intervention or a response, that can be informed by the reflective nature of clinical reasoning. Likewise, the tandem nature of reflection and anticipation in clinical reasoning is reflexively intertwined with informed judgment. Together, clinical judgment and clinical reasoning are essential components of nursing practice and thinking like a nurse (Tanner, 2006).

USING SIMULATIONS TO PROMOTE CLINICAL JUDGMENT

Similar to the clinical arena, advances in technology have greatly impacted educational delivery methods across the educational spectrum beginning in early childhood education and beyond. In many instances, the technology is no longer as cost prohibitive, allowing for the creation of enhanced learning environments that support a diverse array of higher-education pedagogy, including simulation. While the word *simulation* often elicits images of a computerized manikin simulation has moved beyond the mere technological components and has emerged as a true pedagogy of its own (Gaba, 2004). Guided by specific objectives (Gaba, 2004), simulation is the use of one or more typologies in an effort to promote, improve, and/or validate a participant's progression from novice to expert (INASCL Board of Directors, 2011).

There are many different types of simulation. The level of fidelity, or believability, is determined by how closely the environment approaches reality (INASCL Board of Directors, 2011). A variety of modes and models can be deployed singularly or paired in an effort to mimic clinical situations and meet specific learning objectives.

Low-fidelity simulation includes case studies, role playing, and partial task trainers, which offer learners an opportunity to practice a variety of psychomotor skills or cognitive skills. Partial task trainers have been used in nursing since the early 1900s (Herrmann, 2008). Typical examples include IV arms and Foley catheter or central line task trainers.

Moderate-level simulation includes several computerized full-body manikins, computerized partial task trainers, and virtual environments offering increasingly realistic clinical situations. Full-body manikins that offer lung and heart sounds or partial birth simulators are examples of moderate-level simulation.

High-fidelity simulation often includes advanced computerized full-body manikins, the use of standardized patients, or a hybrid that couples one or more of these types of simulations. Recalling that the level of fidelity translates to the believability of the situation rather than the technological sophistication of the equipment, an example might be utilizing a standardized patient in the real clinical environment in a real hospital bed. Usually, high-fidelity simulations usually immerse learners in a more complex, time-sensitive situation requiring specific critical actions, allowing for measurement of clinical reasoning and judgment.

While distance education methodology partners extremely well with some levels of simulation, such as case studies, other levels of simulation, such as hands-on experiences using computerized patients, present many challenges. However, the ability to immerse learners into simulated environments provides situated learning and promotes clinical imagination. Simulated environments can be customized and available 24 hours a day, allowing for a more naturalistic learning process of trial and error and supporting the development of clinical reasoning skills. Additionally, the benefits of learning by doing provide the necessary self-reflection activities needed for higher-order thinking.

Sources of Simulations

Faculty must choose between creating their own simulation scenarios and using ones designed by others. There are pros and cons to both approaches. The major advantage of using predesigned simulations is that it saves time. There are a wide variety of scenarios available from multiple sources, some of which are free. Several publishers create both stand-alone simulation products as well as ones designed to accompany specific textbooks. Manikin manufacturers also create prepackaged scenarios that have usually been peer reviewed and tested. Both of these sources may be expensive and may require ongoing fees or licensures. Another consideration, of particular concern to faculty teaching web courses, is that some supplemental teaching materials from these sources may carry copyright restrictions or may not be formatted to readily share on the web.

Professional or educational organization websites often prove ideal sources for finding predesigned simulation that are frequently free. For instance, the National League for Nursing (2010) currently posts the Advancing Care Excellence for Seniors (ACES) simulation scenarios on their website (www.nln.org/facultyprograms/facultyresources/ACES). These unfolding cases were created to help students learn the evidence-based care of older adults. Cases include simulation templates, instructor tool kits, and charting materials for students that can be shared via the web. The teaching strategy section of Quality and Safety Education for Nurses website (www.QSEN.org) is another source for free predesigned simulation scenarios. However, instructors should be aware that materials from this source vary in completeness, and supplemental materials may need to be reformatted for use in their institution.

One of the potential disadvantages of using prepackaged simulations is the risk of allowing technology to drive the curriculum (Guimond & Salas, 2009). This can happen when simulations are selected based on availability instead of course learning objectives. One solution for this problem is to carefully review the learning objectives and to modify prepackaged scenarios. Jarzemsky, McCarthy, and Ellis (2009) suggest that including aspects from faculty's clinical experiences to these simulations can improve the quality of the learning experience.

The preferred choice for many instructors is to design their own simulations. In one study, 66% of the participants wrote their own scenarios (Sole, Guimond, & Stewart-Amidei, 2011). Some educators enjoy the creativity of the design process and feel that it is the best way to ensure that the learning objectives are addressed. The disadvantage of this practice is that designing scenarios is a time-consuming process that requires faculty training. Unfortunately, too often, instructors are not fully compensated for the time it takes to design and test scenarios (Jeffries, 2008).

The use of a template can facilitate the process of creating a simulation (Jeffries, 2007), and many instructors find that the time it takes to create a scenario decreases with experience. Jeffries (2008) also recommends a team approach to designing and implementing scenarios where team members assume responsibility for various aspects of the project. A consortium approach is another way to create simulation scenarios. For instance, four schools of nursing came together to create and test a simulation-based cardiac assessment curriculum for advanced practice nurses (Jeffries et al., 2011). This approach has many advantages, including the ability to rapidly test and evaluate scenarios. Consortia can also be the sources of predesigned simulations. For instance, the California Maternal Quality Care Collaboration is a source for obstetrical simulations (www.cmqcc.org).

ONLINE, TELEHEALTH, AND BLENDED SIMULATIONS

Providing educational experiences for learners who live in remote areas, perhaps a great distance from the school of nursing, is a challenge that can be met by distance learning. Provision of clinical experiences is more complicated as the student may live a considerable distance from a clinical site, and the number and types of clinical experiences may be limited in some rural areas. Simulation has been viewed as a method to meet some of these clinical instruction challenges. However, even using simulation can be challenging when students and faculty are not at the same location. New variations of distance education incorporate simulation. Simulation using instructor-made videos that demonstrate realistic and relevant scenario-based care is one method. This may be a recording of a high-fidelity simulation using a human patient simulator where either the faculty or other students play the roles. The students can learn vicariously by being the observers to these simulations (Harland, Biddle, & Fallacaro, 2008). Live streaming of a simulation where other students are the active participants and the distance education students are in the role of the observers can also be used. Debriefing for all students could occur via video conferencing.

It is also possible for students to actively participate in a simulation with a human patient simulator when they are at a satellite location with the manikin and the instructor is at a different site controlling the manikin. As the human patient simulators are controlled by a software program, remote desktop control of the computer by a simulation technician is possible. The advantages are that students who live in remote areas can actively experience an identical high-fidelity learning experience as those students able to be on the main campus. Additionally, all students can receive the same type of guidance and feedback from the faculty. A disadvantage is that more than one manikin may be needed (one on the main campus and one at the remote location) and that they would need to be maintained and stored between uses. Another disadvantage is that someone would still be needed at the remote location who can set up the props and set the stage for the simulation before the learners arrive. A potential limitation to the use of remote desktop access may be that the Internet service could have bandwidth problems, causing delays in the simulator's response. "Cloud computing" with IP addresses can help to resolve these issues. Despite potential drawbacks, these experiences have been found to be effective teaching and learning strategies in distance education (Guzic et al., 2011; Medical Readiness Trainer Team, 2001). Point-to-point video teleconferencing increases the value of remote simulation, although students may initially find the technology intimidating (Guzic et al., 2011). More information and technology support are required when point-to-point video teleconferencing is added to the experience.

Grady (2011) describes a unique distance education method for providing a clinical experience for students, which they normally would not be able to experience. She referred to this experience as Virtual Clinical Practicum. Via teleconferencing, students spent several hours at the bedside of a real patient who was in a military hospital several hundred miles from the nursing school. Students observed patient care given by expert nurses. Students were also able to view the role of various team members caring for the patient. Students speaking through microphones were able to verbally interact in "live time" with the nurses, other team members, and the patients and their families during the course of the clinical experience. Built into this experience were break points to allow discussion between the students in a clinical group and their clinical faculty. The use of teleconferencing as a simulated clinical day requires significant planning and coordination. This experience should be piloted prior to going live so that problems can be identified and resolved. A drawback of this type of distance education is that it requires technical support on both sides of the video connection to deliver a smooth experience for students. Video technicians must communicate via phone during the session to correct any sound or video issues. Many technical needs must be met such as sound mix, camera angles, and lighting to maximize the experience. Grady further comments that strong administrative support at both the school and the clinical area was needed for success with this video conferencing simulation. Faculty need to consider the confidentiality issues and guarantee that patient consent is procured for the experience. When some students evaluated this clinical experience, they expressed concern that there was no hands-on component. This could be addressed by the use of a simulation with a human patient simulator. The simulation chosen for that experience should assist the student in applying knowledge learned from the observed clinical day. Due to the time and expense of creating a successful experience with video conference technology, several schools collaborate to create these experiences. Students at multiple sites could then participate simultaneously in the clinical experience.

Video conferencing may have limitations. Taylor (2011) reported that in a small exploratory study, students found that discussion during video conferencing was hampered by several issues. Students reported difficulty seeing and interpreting nonverbal behaviors due to camera angles and the 2-D effect of the videoconference. Students also reported difficulty maintaining eye contact, as they would look at the screen instead of the camera. They would be distracted by their own image on screen. Loss of eye contact with the other person also made it difficult to interpret that person's communication. Students found it difficult to determine if the loss of eye contact was related to the subject matter or related to the technology. Technical issues such as lag times or pauses also caused concern for students, as they had difficulty determining if the other person had or had not completed speaking.

Realism may be more difficult to incorporate during online or distance education than in face-to-face situations, as there can be technical constraints for what is viewed or how it is viewed. An online synchronous discussion forum where faculty could facilitate debriefing via discussion questions may help to overcome this (Rush, Dyches, Waldrop, & Davis, 2008), but it also minimizes the benefits of flexibility that students enjoy with online learning.

A final suggestion for the use of telehealth in nursing education turns the learning upside down. A simulated patient (either a manikin or a standardized patient) can be recorded via telehealth technology. Students would view the patient from a distance, the same way they would during a telehealth session. Nursing students would then practice strategies for using telehealth technologies effectively. The goal would be for them to become practitioners of this technology, not using the technologies for basic knowledge acquisition.

Prerecorded Video Simulation

Incorporating visual components into online learning, such as from a video, adds value to the learning experience. This is because images and words are processed at different sites in the central nervous system, so visualization will enhance learning and recall (Harland et al., 2008). When faculty use a video either as online preparation for a face-to-face simulation or as the actual online simulation, they have the same responsibilities. Faculty must consult with their informational technologists to confirm that their school has the capability to stream the video. Faculty must serve as the content experts for the video. In the case of faculty-created videos, they must likely also become the scriptwriter, producer of the videos, and casting director, who locates actors, either a standardized patient or a fellow faculty member, to portray the roles in the video. Completion of all tasks required for making realistic videos can be quite time consuming. Guhde (2010) reported that the production of three videos for use online that totaled less than 10 minutes of running time required 4 hours. In the first video, an incomplete patient assessment was shown. In the second video, the patient's physiological deterioration was shown as a consequence of improper assessment. In the third video, the complete and accurate assessment was demonstrated. This video included voice-over narration that discussed the aspects of the assessment that were incomplete in the first video and how early detection of a problem or change in a patient's condition could prevent the more serious cascade of events shown in the second video. In the third video, the faculty functioned as the role model and the guide to student learning. Other authors have described the benefit to student learning when faculty assume the role of "a guide on the side" by providing a version of a web-based video or simulation with either a voice-over by faculty explaining the clinical reasoning and expected skills throughout the encounter, or captioned information presented as text under the simulation. In this way, students can confirm that their interpretation of the simulation was correct and complete (Blake & Scanlon, 2007; Hauer et al., 2009).

When faculty use a premade, purchased video, some of the responsibilities for creating the simulation experience are minimized, but faculty still need to carefully review the video to determine its appropriateness for the learner and the learning objectives. A premade video may still require editing to fit the educational goals of the simulation or the needs of the learner.

In Situ Cases Blending With Online Questions

In order to integrate simulation into distance education, some programs require students to participate in learning activities held at designated simulation laboratories (Morrison, Scarcello, Thibeault, & Walker, 2009). As an alternative, distance educators may choose to utilize in situ simulations, or simulations that take place in the clinical environment. In situ simulation is thought to better replicate real-world work flow and offers a mechanism for training and evaluating the entire health care team (Miller, Riley, Davis, & Hansen, 2008; Van Schaik, Plant, Diane, Tsang, & O'Sullivan, 2011). When simulations take place in the workplace, learning can be maximized because participants are already familiar with their environment (Guise et al., 2010). The opportunities and the challenges for the distance educator are building the strong collaborative relations with practice partners that make student participation in such simulations possible.

With in situ simulation, the students still interact with other learners. These learners may be classmates but are just as likely to be other members of the health care team. Thus, in situ simulations are an ideal mechanism to help learners master quality and safety competencies related to teamwork and collaboration (Guise et al., 2010; Miller et al., 2008; Van Schaik et al., 2011). These simulations may also be structured so that the primary interaction is with a standardized patient (Satava, 2009). While simulation centers often have better videotaping capabilities that practice sites, filming patient encounters still may be possible with portable recording devices. Video recordings then may be shared with instructors and used to evaluate the student's skills or the learning experience.

One of the primary disadvantages of using in situ simulations is that there is limited availability of actual clinical sites and scenarios (Gaba, 2004). In situ simulation scenarios are usually designed by the clinical setting to meet the institution's specific training needs. The problem is that while objectives for scenarios used in simulation centers tend to be related to course competencies or proficiencies, objectives for scenarios that occur in situ typically focus on reinforcing skills and identifying deficiencies in the team or clinical systems (Patterson, Blike, & Nadkarni,

2008). Thus, educators must review course and simulation objectives carefully to ensure the best learning experience before assigning student participation. Another challenge to using in situ simulations is that they are frequently canceled at the last minute due to availability of participants or high census or high acuity at the practice site (Patterson et al., 2008). This may leave the educator trying to find last-minute alternative learning experiences for students.

Students may not feel the same level of interaction with their instructor with in situ simulations compared to participating in scenarios at simulation laboratories. Instructors may not be present to support students immediately before or after the learning experience. The use of synchronous or asynchronous online discussions following a simulation is one solution to this problem. The instructor can pose online questions to help students reflect on the experience. This also allows the instructor the opportunity to give students feedback and evaluate their learning.

In the online learning environment, instructors hold the primary role of facilitators who identify learning outcomes, design learning activities, and evaluate student performance (Billings & Halstead, 2009). The instructor's role is much the same when implementing in situ simulations in distance education. The instructor must clearly convey the student's abilities and the learning objectives to the on-site facility to ensure that students are assigned responsibilities consistent with their level of education. They must also coordinate the experience with the practice site, convey the objectives and presimulation assignments to the students, and ensure that learners have the opportunity to reflect on the experience. The use of well-designed online questions can be used to facilitate reflection and evaluate student learning. The role of the learners is to come prepared and to be open to the experience. They should actively participate in the simulation, the immediate debriefing on site, and the subsequent debriefing with the instructor.

Sources

In situ simulations are often created by an institution to rehearse and improve team responses to high-risk situations (Patterson et al., 2008). Scenarios are sometimes created to mimic a clinical situation that occurred in the facility or may be created to test a system's resources to address specific problems. In situ simulations may be designed to use either manikins or standardized patients (Gaba, 2004; Satava, 2009). Mobile simulation units may also be used to implement in situ simulations. For instance, Guise et al. (2008) created a mobile obstetrical simulation unit that traveled among rural and community hospitals to provide standardized training in obstetrical emergencies. The providers felt that this type of program proved an effective way to learn and maintain infrequently used obstetrical skills and uncover safety problems. Instructors with experience in simulation design can collaborate with practice institutions to help them to design scenarios that incorporate best educational principles.

Due to time constraints in the practice setting, in situ simulations must be concise. Empty rooms used for a scenario may need to be filled with a patient at a moment's notice, and no alternative space may be available on the practice unit to engage in postsimulation discussion. Thus, debriefing may be especially challenging. One facility reported limiting in situ simulations to 10 minutes and the debriefing to 7 minutes due to time and resource limitations (Patterson et al., 2008). While an on-site facilitator may lead the initial debriefing, it is critically important that the distance educator puts in place a mechanism to ensure that students engage in reflection. This again can be accomplished through online discussions.

EXAMPLES OF UNFOLDING SIMULATIONS IN AN ONLINE ENVIRONMENT

Unfolding simulation cases evolve over time in an unpredictable manner. A few approaches to an unfolding case may include three to four events that build upon each other, providing students a view across a clinical event, a hospitalization, or the life span (Page, Kowlowitz, & Alden, 2010). Purposes of unfolding cases vary, but a few include the following:

1. They demonstrate hierarchal order so the learner can view the health disruption progression and symptom management; for example, the first case demonstrates the patient being admitted with head injury due to a fall and requiring a focused neurological assessment. The unfolding case leads to the second scenario where the patient experiences specific neurological signs, for example, severe headache, widening pulse pressure, and so forth. The third case is post craniotomy, where the patient requires care after removal of the subdural hematoma.
2. They help visualize and prioritize hospital trajectory and care of a patient that progresses. For example, the patient is admitted

through the emergency department, with the learner performing an assessment. In the second scenario, the patient is admitted to the progressive care unit, and the learner is to provide the assessment and care needed in this setting. In the third unfolding case, the patient is ready for discharge, and the learner must provide the appropriate discharge instructions.

3. They provide the learner a view across the patient's life span showing an impact of the health disruption/disease process and nursing interventions required. The first case depicts a newly diagnosed patient with acute renal failure (ARF). The second case shows the patient with compromised acid/base balance related to ARF. The third case depicts the same patient with end-stage disease requiring end-of-life care.
4. They serve as a mechanism to include a variety of important assessments/findings where one event leads to another. For example, the first case focuses on a patient with hypotension and subtle findings of sepsis. In the second, case the patient is now critically ill with sepsis and hypotension.

Several organizations have developed unfolding case studies related to particular topics, which are available at no cost to faculty. Four unfolding cases that focus on older adults and address the complexity of decision making related to their care can be found at www.nln.org/facultydevelopment/facultyresources/ACES/index.htm. Unfolding cases related to patient safety can be found at the Quality and Safety Education for Nursing site at www.qsen.org. Unfolding cases can be videotaped with students observing them in a distance-education environment. Following viewing of the cases, use of a discussion forums, a wiki, or a VoiceThread™ can provide debriefing for the learner.

USING EMERGING TECHNOLOGIES FOR SIMULATION (SECOND LIFE AND SIMULATORS)

In this section, different types of emerging technologies (for example, Second Life, simulations, and other types of technologies) will be described as new teaching methods for educators to use when teaching nursing students enrolled in distance education courses. Examples of different educational methodologies will be discussed in addition to considerations to think about when incorporating technology-type activities into distance education courses.

TABLE 8.1 Considerations to Address When Incorporating Second Life Into a Required Nursing Course

1. The use of Second Life as a teaching tool requires detailed planning for technology and for the experience. Orientation for all faculty and students is critical.
2. Strong technological support is essential so that faculty can focus on the education and instructional technologists can focus on functionality.
3. Initial scheduling for students, the technical team, and equipment is time consuming, but after experience, time requirements for scheduling become streamlined.
4. A review of the course concepts can reveal where the online activities best fit in the overall course, for example, as a prerequisite to real clinical experiences.
5. Avatar nurses and patients can effectively produce realistic interview sessions. These experiences can provide student nurses with experience with a diverse group of patients.
6. Second Life can be designed as a sound educational strategy to prepare for clinical experiences or reinforce clinical concepts. Its use overcomes barriers between classroom and clinical teaching.

Adapted from Sweigart, Hodson-Carlton, Campbell, Lutz, & Thede (2010).

Sweigart, Hodson-Carlton, Campbell, Lutz, and Thede (2010) incorporated Second Life into their teaching both in face-to-face classrooms and via distance education course activities. After implementing their virtual activities using Second Life to provide interview skills and development of teaching plans for the assigned patients, the authors developed a set of lessons learned to consider the effectiveness of their teaching methodologies. The considerations from their educational exploration, when incorporating emerging technologies into a distance-education nursing course, are displayed in Table 8.1.

Exemplars of Interaction Using Emerging Technologies Via Second Life and Simulations

Stewart et al. (2010) developed the use of virtual reality and integrated the activities into their BSN degree nursing program. Second Life, developed by Linden Lab of San Francisco, California (www.secondlife.com), is a freely available online virtual world that can be used in simulations. A virtual world is a computer-based simulated environment in a 3-D format where multiple users can interact and communicate with one another. Participants are represented in an avatar, which is a humanoid form. Moving through the virtual environment to manipulate objects, performing assessments, and communicating with others through instant messaging are all methods of activity demonstrated by the avatars. One of the initial steps for instructional designers was to establish a physical presence in Second Life by creating a place to meet; hence, the builder developed a virtual campus. The first building constructed was the anchor building representing an alumni house on campus. Office space was also created for faculty so the students could have office hours with the faculty as needed. When developing the Second Life activities, the developers created a Student Leadership Team (SLT) to provide ongoing feedback to administrators and faculty for improving the quality of the students' experience in the nursing program. The team consisted of six different students and two student service coordinators who meet as avatars and have voice chat to discuss issues, concerns, and new ideas.

EXAMPLES OF USING SECOND LIFE IN A DISTANCE EDUCATION FORMAT

Community Health

On the Midwest campus, Stewart et al. (2010) reported that Second Life developers and faculty met as a team to discuss how community health nursing could be experienced in a Second Life environment due to the lack of experienced public health nurses and the challenge of finding safe, quality community healthy sites. Using the Essential Public Health Service list from the U.S. Centers for Disease Control and Prevention as a framework, the Second Life activities were created to achieve these critical public health issues and nursing roles in this specialty. For example, each public health office was designed to open to a central courtyard. One student assignment was to visit the Women's, Infants, and Children's (WIC) office, which has various links to other health offices. These links help students realize all the services for which the office is accountable. Students, through their avatars, observe a nutrition interview of a simulated WIC client. Another example was a student's visit to inspect areas in a restaurant looking for health and sanitation issues. The avatar could teleport to the restaurant, conduct the screening, and then develop a report, serving as the inspector, and send to the instructor. All the scenarios created in the virtual world were embedded with a case study and a lecture that was also provided online.

Postclinical Conferences

Second Life experiences have also become a forum for conducting postclinical conferences. Initially, these conferences were held in a learning management system with chat sessions conducted by the faculty to address questions and to communicate issues/concerns to students. Although useful information was shared between and among faculty and students, looking at the screen with type print moving across, students felt that the experience was impersonal. In Second Life, students now meet in a designated gathering place where the instructor moderates the chat with voice while the students use text messaging. This type of communication allows more time for students to interject questions and to share great clinical learning experiences (Stewart et al., 2010).

Mental Health Nursing

Students in a mental health nursing course need to understand schizophrenia and the impact of the disease on a patient's life. To address these needs, faculty from the University of California–Davis provide students with an experiential learning activity in Second Life. To help students understand the incessant and powerful nature of the voices heard by patients with schizophrenia, the faculty used virtual hallucinations. As students enter the Second Life world, an MP3 voice file begins to play. Students have reflected on how realistic and informative the experiences are to hear—they are very insightful, scary, and terrible as described by the learners. In addition to the learning experiences, students are encouraged to attend support groups in Second Life for depression, bipolar disorder, and substance abuse (Stewart et al., 2010).

Nutritional Assessment in a Physical-Assessment Course

Sweigart et al. (2010) developed a Second Life nutritional assessment experience that was a required activity for a health assessment course. Nursing faculty developed 20 standardized clients from ages 17 to 82 years representing four different ethnic groups. Scenarios for the virtual patients were similar to those witnessed in real-life experiences. To conduct assessments, students had to travel to a virtual clinic where, using their own avatars, they interviewed patients in Second Life who were trained volunteers playing the part of a standardized client. Students used a screening tool "Determine Your Nutritional Health" approved by the American Academy of Family Physicians, American Dietetic Association, and National Council of the Aging, Inc. Clients completed the screening instrument—name, occupation, and so forth—in the lobby of the virtual clinic. This information was provided to the student nurse interviewer as a foundation for the interview. The comprehensive interview was then conducted using private messaging. The captured interview transcript allowed students an opportunity to reflect and self-critique their interviewing skills.

Second Life applications have also provided virtual clinical experiences for nursing students who are in high-risk situations and ones that rarely occur, like disaster scenarios (Schmidt & Stewart, 2009; Schmidt & Stewart, 2010; Stewart, Pope, & Duncan, 2009).

STUDENT-DIRECTED SCENARIOS

Another potential method of using simulations via distance learning was demonstrated by Schwartz, Green, and Faser (2010). These educators used the Classroom Performance System (CPS) by eInstruction to give quizzes and tests and record attendance. This system uses a response pad, commonly referred to as a "clicker," which allows the students to electronically register answers to questions. In a database, the answers are recorded and can be immediately analyzed to assess student understanding of concepts and material. The ability to use this system enabled faculty to transform a few of their simulations into student-directed outcome scenarios. The simulation scenario videos are shown in class or in a distance education course, students see the video snippet online, and then the students are asked to choose an ending for the scenario with their clickers. For example, if students are watching care of the postthoracotomy patient, and there is fluctuation of fluid in the underwater seal chamber of the pleurovac, the camera pans to the patient's vital signs, in addition to showing the nurse asking the patient questions. At this point, the video is paused while the instructor asks the class a multiple-choice question about the appropriate nursing response. The question and response from the class are shown on the screen for students to select the correct answer using their clickers. The responses are tracked, and then the video is continued so the students can see the appropriate nursing intervention. The use of CPS within the scenario has received high praise from the students. This teaching–learning activity, as described, could be used in a large classroom setting as discussed, or video snippets can be inserted in a web-based course, with students viewing the video and then selecting an answer in an embedded learning activity about the video.

The future direction of nursing education will include additional use of these new technological activities as the technical consciousness of faculty continue to increase. With today's creative and technologically advanced students, nursing faculty must be committed to exploring and implementing new ways to engage students in their learning.

DEBRIEFING THE DISTANCE LEARNER

Debriefing is the period at the end of a simulated clinical encounter when the faculty and student re-examine the experience (Dreifuerst, 2009). Debriefing can be a structured or unstructured process. Debriefing provides an opportunity for students and faculty to re-examine what occurred during the simulation process and discern what has been learned. Nursing faculty generally focus the discussion or activities on learning outcomes and the intended objectives of the experience (Fuller, 2007). Debriefing can include reflective practice when students analyze their own assumptions and actions to think about how to further enhance or develop more skillful nursing practice (Decker, 2007).

When debriefing is used as a reflective learning opportunity, faculty and students engage in recollection, review, reflection, and analysis of the events of the simulation and the thinking processes of the student(s) during the simulation experience (Dreifuerst, 2009). Reflection is a component of metacognition. It can occur both during and after clinical experiences through reflection in action and reflection on action (Schön, 1983). Reflective practitioners who engage in introspection learn to self-correct and assimilate new experiences with prior ones and thus improve professional competence (Rudolph, Simon, Rivard, Dufresne, & Raemer, 2007). In addition, when skills in reflection are facilitated through debriefing, students learn to embed this into their nursing practice and develop clinical reasoning and clinical judgment (Dreifuerst, 2010).

Facilitating debriefing is an important faculty role when teaching distance education students. The narrative recounting and analysis of the clinical experience can take many different formats. Synchronous dialog through voice and video over Internet programs is an option that allows for group or individual discussion to occur in real time. Conversely, asynchronous activities could include viewing video of the simulation, posting on group discussion boards, blog concept mapping, and reflective journaling. Regardless of the method, faculty feedback regarding both the simulation experience and the reflection is an important piece of the learning environment. It is critical for faculty to debrief student clinical experiences with the distance learner. The use of open-ended questions is an established technique that can be used in any learning environment to guide the reflection and facilitate the debriefing process (Arafeh, Hansen, & Nichols, 2010). There is increasing evidence in the literature that debriefing is essential for learning in simulation pedagogy (Shinnick, Woo, Horwich, & Steadman, 2011). Using creative strategies for engaging distance learners in group reflection and dialog can provide an opportunity for the student to construct knowledge and to test it against the ideas and knowledge of other students. This reflective knowledge provides the foundation for clinical reasoning and judgment.

SUMMARY AND KEY POINTS

The future of nursing education is here, with new technologies being used in both face-to-face classroom and clinical settings as well as in distance education learning platforms. In nursing education, traditional current teaching and learning practices may not always facilitate the development of clinical reasoning at the level needed for nursing graduates. Both modalities must be restructured to provide the student with opportunities to learn clinical reasoning and judgment. There are a variety of approaches to teaching nursing students clinical reasoning/clinical judgment that can be utilized as highlighted in this chapter. Faculty need to be committed to engaging students in learning the nursing knowledge and skills required to be a competent, safe practitioner. Today's students are creative, technologically savvy, and advanced in their technology skills set. Nursing education must capture the students' creativity and imagination and inspire them to understand real-life health care and patient expectations. Nursing education must develop new ways to improve the critical judgment and reasoning of nursing graduates in order to ultimately improve patient care.

REFERENCES

Aiken, L., Clarke, S., Cheung, R., Sloane, D., & Silber, J. (2003). Educational levels of hospital nurses and surgical patient mortality. *JAMA: Journal of the American Medical Association, 290*(12), 1617–1623.

American Association of Colleges of Nursing. (1998). *The essentials of baccalaureate education for professional nursing practice.* Washington DC: Author.

Arafeh, J. M., Hansen, S. S., & Nichols, A. (2010). Debriefing in simulated-based learning: Facilitating a reflective discussion. *Journal of Perinatal & Neonatal Nursing, 24*(4), 302–309, quiz 310–301.

Benner, P. (1984). *From novice to expert: Excellence and power in clinical nursing practice.* Menlo Park, CA: Addison-Wesley.

Billings, D. M., & Halstead, J. A. (2009). *Teaching and learning in nursing* (3rd Ed.). St. Louis, MO: Saunders.

Blake, C., & Scanlon, E. (2007). Reconsidering simulations in science education at a distance: Features of effective use. *Journal of Computer Assisted Learning*, 23, 491–502.

Chaffin, A. J., & Maddux, C. D. (2004). Internet teaching methods for use in baccalaureate nursing education. *CIN: Computers, Informatics, Nursing, 22*(3), 132–142.

Childs, J. C., & Sepples, S. (2006). Clinical teaching by simulation: Lessons learned from a complex patient care scenario. *Nursing Education Perspectives, 27*(3), 154–158.

Decker, S. (2007). Integrating guided reflection into simulated learning experiences. In P. Jeffries (Ed.), *Simulation in Nursing* (pp. 21–33). New York, NY: National League for Nursing.

Dowding, D., & Thompson, C. (2003). Measuring the quality of judgment and decision-making in nursing. *Journal of Advanced Nursing, 44*(1), 49–57.

Dreifuerst, K. T. (2009). The essentials of debriefing in simulation learning: A concept analysis. *Nursing Education Perspectives, 30*(2), 109–114.

Dreifuerst, K. T. (2010). *Debriefing for meaningful learning: Fostering development of clinical reasoning through simulation* (Doctoral dissertation, Indiana University Scholar Works Repository). Retrieved from Dissertations and Theses, http://hdl.handle.net/1805/2459

Dreyfus, H. L., & Dreyfus, S. E. (1986). *Mind over machine: The power of human intuition and expertise in the era of the computer*. New York, NY: The Free Press.

Ebright, P. R., Patterson, E. S., Chalko, B. A., & Render, M. L. (2003). Understanding the complexity of registered nurse work in acute care settings. *Journal of Nursing Administration, 33*(12), 630–638.

Facione, N. C., & Facione, P. A. (2008). Critical thinking and clinical judgment. In N. C. Facione & P. A. Facione (Eds.), *Critical thinking and clinical reasoning in the health sciences* (pp. 1–13). Millbrae, CA: California Academic Press.

Fuller, M. (2007). Theoretical framework for simulation design. In P. Jeffries (Ed.). *Simulation in nursing* (pp. 21–33). New York, NY: National League for Nursing.

Gaba, D. M. (2004). The future vision of simulation in health care. *Quality and Safety in Health Care, 13*(Suppl 1) i2–i10. doi:10.1136/qshc.2004.009878

Grady, J. L. (2011) The Virtual Clinical Practicum: An innovative telehealth model for clinical nursing education. *Nursing Education Perspectives*, 32 (3), 189–194.

Guhde, J. (2010). Clinical decision-making: Using online exercises and patient simulation to improve students' clinical decision-making. *Nursing Education Perspectives, 31*(6), 387–389. doi:10.1043/1536-5026-31.6.387

Guimond, M. E., & Salas, E. (2009). Linking the science of training to nursing simulation. *Nurse Educator, 34*(3). 105–106. doi:10.1097/NNE.0b013e31819fb305

Guise, J. M., Lowe, N. K., Deering, S., Lewis, P. O., O'Haire, C., Irwin, L. K., Kanki, B. G. (2008). Mobile in situ obstetric emergency simulation and teamwork training to improve maternal–fetal safety in hospitals. *Joint Commission Journal on Quality and Patient Safety, 36*(10), 443–453.

Guzic, B. L., McIlhenny, C. V., Knee, D. R., LeMoine, J. K., Wendekier, C. M., Demuth, B. R., Bapat, A. (2011). Distance learning and clinical simulation in senior baccalaureate nursing education. *Clinical Simulation in Nursing, 7*(5), 000–000. doi:10.1016/j.ecns.2011.04.005

Harland, W., Biddle, C., & Fallacaro, M. (2008). Audiovisual facilitation of clinical knowledge: a paradigm for dispersed student education based on Paivio's Dual Coding Theory. *American Association of Nurse Anesthetists Journal, 76*(3), 194–198.

Hauer, K. E., Chou, C. L., Souza, K. H., Henry, D., Loeser, H., Burke, C., & O'Sullivan, P. (2009). Impact of an in-person versus web-based practice standardized patient examination on student performance on a subsequent high-stakes standardized patient examination. *Teaching & Learning in Medicine, 21*(4), 284–290. doi:10.1080/10401330903228307

Herrmann, E. K. (2008). Remembering Mrs. Chase. Before there were Smart Hospitals and Sim-Men, there was "Mrs. Chase." *Imprint, 55*(2), 52–55.

Higgs, J., & Jones, M. A. (2008). Clinical decision making and multiple problem spaces. In J. Higgs, M. A. Jones, S. Loftus, & N. Christenson (Eds.), *Clinical Reasoning in the health professions* (p. 3-17). London, England: Elsevier.

INASCL Board of Directors. (2011). Standard I: Terminology. *Clinical Simulation in Nursing, 7*(4S), s3–7. doi:10.1016/j.ecns.2011.05.005

Jarzemsky, P. M., McCarthy, J., & Ellis, N. (2009). Incorporating quality and safety education for nurses competencies in simulation scenario design. *Nurse Educator, 34*(3), 105–106. doi:10.1097/NNE.0b013e31819fb305

Jeffries, P. R. (2007). *Simulation in nursing education from conceptualization to evaluation.* New York, NY: National League for Nursing.

Jeffries, P. R. (2008). Getting in S.T.E.P. with simulations: Simulations take educator preparation. *Nursing Education Perspectives, 29*(2), 70–73.

Jeffries, P. R., Beach, M., Decker, S. I., Dlugasch, L., Groom, G., Settles, J., & O'Donnell, J. M. (2011). Multi-center development and testing of a simulation-based cardiovascular assessment curriculum for advanced practice nurses. *Nursing Education Perspectives, 32*(5), 316–322. doi:10.5480/1536-5026-32.5.316SJe

Kane, R., Sandretto, S., & Heath, C. (2004). An investigation into excellent tertiary teaching: Emphasising reflective practice. *Higher Education, 47*(3), 283–310. doi:10.1023/b:high.0000016442.55338.24

Klein, G. (1999) *Sources of power: How people make decisions*. Cambridge, MA: MIT Press.

Larew, C., Lessans, S., Spunt, D., Foster, D., & Covington, B. G. (2006). Innovations in clinical simulation: Application of Benner's theory in an interactive patient care simulation. *Nursing Education Perspectives, 27*(1), 16–21.

Lasater, K. (2007). Clinical judgment development: Using simulation to create an assessment rubric. *Journal of Nursing Education, 46*(11), 496–503.

Levett-Jones, T. L., Hoffman, K. A., Dempsey, J., Jeong, Y.-S., Noble, D. I., Norton, C. A., Roche, J. M., Hickey, N. (2010). 'The 'five rights' of clinical reasoning: An educational model to enhance nursing students' ability to identify and manage clinically 'at risk' patients', *Nurse Education Today, 30*(6), 515–520.

Miller, K., Riley, W., Davis, S., & Hansen, H. (2008). In situ simulation: A method of experiential learning to promote safety and team behavior. *Journal of Perinatal & Neonatal Nursing, 22*(2), 105–113. doi:10.1097/01.JPN.0000319096.97790.f7

Morrison, B., Scarcello, M., Thibeault, L., & Walker, D. (2009). The use of a simulated nursing practice lab in a distance practical nursing program. *Clinical Simulation in Nursing, 5*(2), e67–e71. doi:10.1016/j.ecns.2009.01.004

National League for Nursing. (2010). *ACES Advancing Care Excellence for Seniors*. Retrieved October 31, 2011, from http://www.nln.org/facultydevelopment/facultyresources/aces/unfolding_cases.htm

Page, J. B., Kowlowitz, V., & Alden, K. R. (2010). Development of a scripted unfolding case. Study focusing on delirium in older adults. *Journal of Continuing Education in Nursing, 41*(5), 225–230.

Patterson, M. D., Blike, G. T, & Nadkarni, V. M. (2008). In situ simulation: Challenges and results. *Advances in Patient Safety: New Directions and Alternative Approaches, 3.* Retrieved from http://www.ahrq.gov/downloads/pub/advances2/vol3/Advances-Patterson_48.pdf

Rhodes M. L., & Curran C. (2005). Use of the human patient simulator to teach clinical judgment skills in a baccalaureate nursing program. *Computers, Informatics, Nursing, 23*(5), 256–262, quiz 263–264. PubMed PMID: 16166827.

Rudolph, J. W., Simon, R., Rivard, P., Dufresne, R. L., & Raemer, D. B. (2007). Debriefing with good judgment: Combining rigorous feedback with genuine inquiry. *Anesthesiology Clinics, 25*(2), 361–376.

Rush, K. L., Dyches, C. E., Waldrop, S., & Davis, A. (2008). Critical thinking among RN-to-BSN distance students participating in human patient simulation. *Journal of Nursing Education, 47*(11), 501–507.

Satava, R. M. (2009).The revolution in medical education—The role of simulation. *Journal of Graduate Medical Education, 1*(2), 172–175. doi:10.4300/JGME-D-09-00075.1

Schmidt, B., & Stewart, S. (2009). Implementing the virtual reality learning environment Second Life. *Nurse Educator, 34*(4), 152–155.

Schmidt, B., & Stewart, S. (2010). Implementing the virtual world of Second Life into community nursing theory and clinical courses. *Nurse Educator, 35*(2), 74–78.

Schön, D. A. (1983). *The reflective practitioner: How professionals think in action.* New York, NY: Basic Books.

Schwartz, M., Green, B., & Faser, K (2010). The digital frontier: Broadcasting simulations for nursing education. *Computers, Informatics, Nursing, 28*(5), 250–253.

Second Life. (2011). *What is Second Life?* Retrieved from http://secondlife.com/whatis/?lang=en-US#Education_&_Enterprise

Shinnick, M. A., Woo, M., Horwich, T. B., & Steadman, R. (2011). Debriefing: The most important component in simulation? *Clinical Simulation in Nursing, 7*(3), e105–e111. doi:10.1016/j.ecns.2010.11.005

Sole, M. L., Guimond, M. E., & Stewart-Amidei, C. (2011). *Instructor simulation resources and needs: A statewide perspective from Florida* [Abstract]. Presented at the Sigma Theta Tau International Conference. Retrieved from http://hdl.handle.net/10755/152779

Stewart, S., Hansen, T., Pope, D., Schmidt, B., Thyes, J., Jayalakshmi, J., & Berthold, T. (2010). Developing a Second Life campus for online accelerated BSN students. *Computers, Informatics, Nursing, 28*(5), 253–258.

Stewart, S., Pope, D., & Duncan, D. (2009).Using Second Life to enhance ACCEL an online accelerated nursing BSN program. *Studies in Health Technology and Informatics, 146*, 636–640.

Sweigart, L., Hodson-Carlton, K., Campbell, B., Lutz, D., & Thede, L. (2010). Second Life environment: A venue for interview skill development. *Computers, Informatics, in Nursing, 28*(5), 258–263.

Tanner, C. A. (2006). Thinking like a nurse: A research-based model of clinical judgment in nursing. *Journal of Nursing Education, 45*(6), 204–211.

Tanner C. A., Padrick, K. P., Westfall, U. E., & Putzier, D. J. (1987). Diagnostic reasoning strategies of nurses and nursing students. *Nursing Research, 36*(6), 358–63. PubMed PMID: 3671123.

Taylor, T. (2011). Video conferencing vs talking face to face: Is video suitable for supportive dialogue? *International Journal of Therapy and Rehabilitation, 18*(7), 392–403.

Teekman, B. (2000). Exploring reflective thinking in nursing practice. *Journal of Advanced Nursing, 31*(5), 1125–1135.

Van Schaik, S. M., Plant, J., Diane, S., Tsang, L., & O'Sullivan, P. (2011). Interprofessional team training in pediatric resuscitation: a low-cost, in situ simulation program that enhances self-efficacy among participants. *Clinical Pediatrics, 50*(9), 807–815.

NINE

Designing Online Learning Activities

DEBORAH J. CLARK

Designing online activities and assignments can be as complex or as simple as nurse educators desire. The types of assignments and learning activities are limited only by the technologies available and the imagination of the course designer/instructor. Sometimes ideas can be stimulated by looking at learning activities designed by colleagues in a nursing program or by nursing faculty at other colleges or universities. Examining learning activities developed by teachers in other disciplines can also bring to mind creative applications in nursing. Many educators like to apply new technology in their distance education classes to add interest and challenges for students.

LAY THE FOUNDATION: PROGRAM AND COURSE OUTCOMES

The goal of any learning activity is to enhance certain types of thinking and reasoning abilities so that students are able to meet the course and program outcomes. In addition to a review of outcomes, nurse educators might consider several questions to stimulate their own imaginations. "What should the student to be able to do at the completion of the course? How can the students demonstrate what they learned? What tangible object would represent achievement of the course objectives?"

Bloom's Taxonomy (and its subsequent revisions) has been used by nurse educators in classroom instruction for many years. This taxonomy is still relevant and can be examined in light of opportunities to craft activities to achieve learning outcomes. The Iowa State University Center for Excellence in Teaching and Learning (2012) has an interactive website (www.celt.iastate.edu/teaching/RevisedBlooms1.html) that nurse educators can use to explore a variety of simple objectives (that can be translated into activities and assignments) at each level of the taxonomy. By simply hovering over a colored block on the taxonomy matrix, educators can see sample activities for the level of expected learning. Using this tool can help nurse educators select tangible outcomes as evidence of achieving certain course or program outcomes.

KNOW THE STUDENTS

A learning activity will be more successful if it is designed with the students' knowledge and abilities in mind. If educators have taught a particular class before, they may have a good idea of the knowledge the students already bring into the class and of expected course outcomes. However, educators developing a new course will need to discover students' knowledge before creating engaging assignments. Collaboration with faculty peers who have taught prerequisite courses may be helpful. Likewise, a review of standards, such as *Essentials of Baccalaureate Education* (AACN, 2008), state board regulations, and National Council Licensure Exam for Registered Nurses (NCLEX-RN®) test blueprints, and other documents can keep educators focused on critical concepts to be developed in online courses.

Certainly, all levels of nursing can discuss the same topic, but the expectations for a tangible assignment or learning activity will be different for each group. For example, in an associate degree program, there may be a unit of study on nursing ethics in the first semester of the program. The students in the course are freshmen, have no prior nursing experience, and may or may not have had a course in ethics or philosophy. The discussions and assignments regarding ethics will necessarily be foundational—knowledge and comprehension, discussions with possibly some application to nursing practice in very basic ways tied to the past experiences of the student in the health care community. However, senior baccalaureate students nearing graduation should have a bit of experience with ethics and ethical dilemmas during clinical and classroom learning. This group of seniors would necessitate a more complex discussion, application, and evaluation of ethics to nursing practice because of their preparation and learning needs. Graduate students, possibly already nurse leaders in their communities, will have a need to understand ethics from a different perspective and apply a range of ethical theories to solve current and future health care problems, improve patient safety, and evaluate outcomes.

It is also necessary to consider the technological preparation of learners and resources available to them. Nurse educators should consider several key questions: (a) Are students novices with computers and technology or more advanced than the educator? (b) Do students have sufficient funds to pay out of pocket for an application, or is there a free alternative? (c) Are any students using dial-up Internet access? (d) How would the learning activity be experienced with bandwidth limitations? If a nursing program has specified certain minimum computer competencies and technology resources, this assessment of students is made much easier.

ASSESS AVAILABLE RESOURCES

As discussed in an earlier chapter, there are many existing materials (learning objectives, apps, and websites with interactive activities) that can be adapted for online nursing classes. Textbook publishers' websites sometimes have electronic learning activities already developed that can be adapted for use as engaging and meaningful activities to encourage clinical reasoning. Some colleges and universities have teaching/learning centers whose missions are to encourage the best practices in undergraduate and graduate education. These centers could have useful resources for nurse educators who are developing online learning activities. Other colleges might place a teaching center in their libraries.

Online resources for instructional technology are readily available for nurse educators. Bloomin' Google (Schrock, 2011) is a website where ideas of available technology for inclusion in distance education courses are cataloged. NovEx (2011) is a website that provides interactive case studies designed to meet the mandates of transformation in nursing education for nursing programs for a per-class student fee. Depending on the program, this may be a feasible and constructive option for faculty and students. The MERLOT Health Sciences Portal offers a number of free, online-peer-reviewed, interactive learning objects and cases that can be easily applied in the distance education class (MERLOT, 2011). Regardless of the source, selecting good-quality activities that assist students in achieving learning outcomes is the goal. Table 9.1 provides additional resources for a nurse educator to locate instructional activities online.

SELECT THE RIGHT TECHNOLOGY

Hixon, Buckenmeyer, and Zamojski (2011) created Bloom's Technology Wheel (Figure 9.1) to help faculty select technology to match their

TABLE 9.1 Instructional Activities

Technology	Article/Author/Website Title	URL
Concept maps	The Theory Underlying Concept Maps and How to Construct Them (Novak & Cañas, 2008)	cmap.ihmc.us/Publications/ResearchPapers/TheoryUnderlyingConceptMaps.pdf
	How to Make a Concept Map in Microsoft Word (eHow, 2011)	www.ehow.com/how_4927645_make-concept-map-microsoft-word.html
	Gliffy—five free concept maps	www.gliffy.com
Crossword puzzles	Instant Online Crossword Puzzle Maker (free)	www.puzzle-maker.com/CW
	Eclipse Crossword (free)	www.eclipsecrossword.com
Photo collage	Google Images	www.google.com (select images)
	Pictures.com	pictures.com
	Independent photos taken by the students	
Blogging	Google Blogger (free)	www.blogger.com
	Wordpress (free)	wordpress.com
	FreeBloggit (free)	freeblogit.com
Videos	YouTube—create your own channel for students to upload their videos	
Surveys	Zoomerang	www.zoomerang.com
	SurveyMonkey	www.surveymonkey.com
Case Studies	How to Write a Case Study (Jeffries, 2011)	www.nursingsociety.org/Education/CourseAdoption/Documents/online_howto.pdf
	National Center for Case Study Teaching in Science	sciencecases.lib.buffalo.edu/cs/

needs and the course objectives. The innermost black circle on the wheel is Bloom's Revised Taxonomy for knowledge, comprehension, application, analysis, synthesis, and evaluation. Connected to this is the next gray ring in the wheel, which provides common verbs used in an objective or outcome for the class. The third ring on the wheel (light gray) represents tangible evidence of achievement of the objective. Supporting this is a fourth ring (dark gray) that labels the different technologies available that can assist students in producing evidence of learning.

EXAMPLES

Using the wheel of Hixon et al. (2011), an instructor who has a course objective that states that "the student will compare and contrast two foreign countries' health care systems" can begin in the analysis level (black ring). The instructor has a variety of tangible assignments (light gray ring) from which to choose: report, model, argument breakdown, and questionnaire. The technology (dark gray ring) that might be used by students in achieving the outcome includes spreadsheets, concept maps, survey tools, and graphing programs. With technology, educators are no longer limited to tests and papers. For example, a concept map could be used to analyze differences and similarities in health care

FIGURE 9.1 Bloom's Technology Wheel

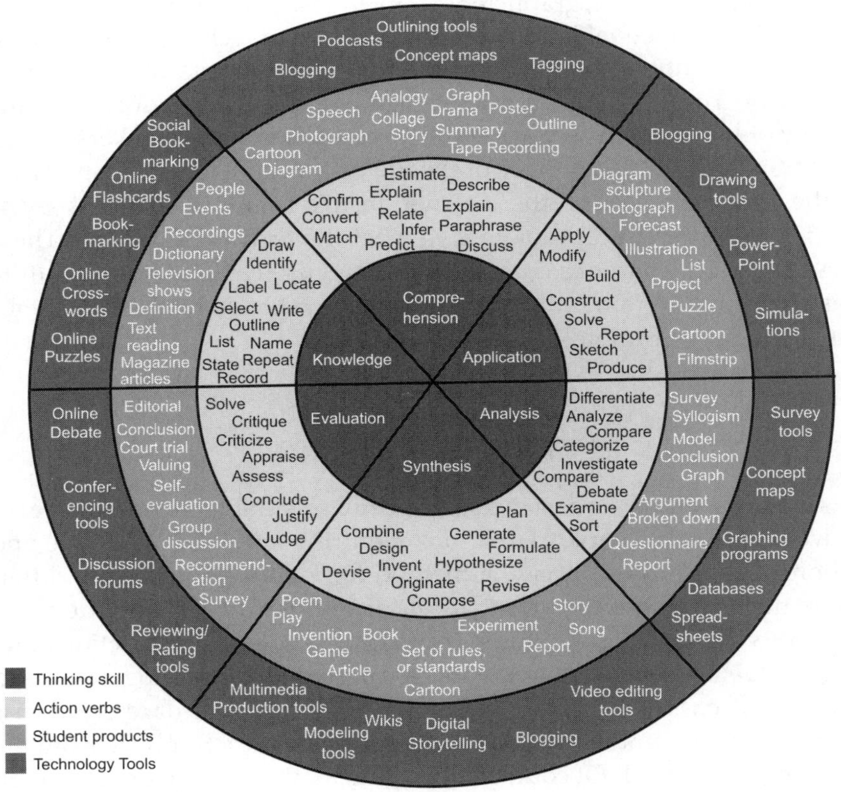

Source: Graphic created by Emily Hixon, Janet Buckenmeyer, and Heather Zamojski, Copyright 2011. Reprinted with permission of the authors. Adapted from a graphic originally published at cstep.csumb.edu/Obj_tutorial/bloomwheel.html (link no longer active).

systems in two countries. The concept map can be drawn using software and saved in a readable format for others to view in an online class. Online discussions can then center on analyses made by all students in the class.

Example for a Nursing Doctoral Program

Doctoral programs often require a written review of literature, extensive papers, and reading assignments. Within assignments are challenges such as organizing a large amount of material, analyzing gaps, summarizing current knowledge, and evaluating a body of work. How might an assignment take advantage of new technologies, add interest for the learners, and produce a sharable, scholarly product? Using the wheel, the "analysis" section shows possible tangible outcomes including (but not limited to) a model, graph, report, and questionnaire (versus the standard written review of literature). Many different technologies could be used by the student to meet this objective. For example, students could create a matrix of critiqued articles using Microsoft® Excel®, document the review of literature in a PowerPoint® presentation with speaker's notes, and prepare an oral summary of the literature using a podcast playable in the online class or on the Internet. In this example, students leveraged three different technologies to meet the learning outcome. These files can become part of a course archive and used as examples in future classes or for program evaluation or could be retained by the student for use during dissertation.

Example for a Graduate Program

Case study methods are particularly useful in nursing as students learn to work through complex situations requiring specific knowledge and actions. Case studies provide a method for faculty to introduce different patient situations in varying levels of complexity and provide a safe structure for students to study, respond, and discuss the actions and knowledge needed to solve the issues presented. Unfolding case studies were discussed in previous chapters, and examples of refereed case studies can be found at the National Center for Case Study Teaching in Science or MERLOT. Of course, nurse educators may also develop their own case studies specific to a course and its course objectives. An additional reference (Flippin, 2010) can be read online before constructing a case study.

One such case study (Rejman, 2010) for nurse practitioner students can be found at the National Center for Case Study Teaching. The case study involves a pregnant female who is not meeting appointments or normal prenatal testing goals. The nurse practitioner is concerned about the patient and discusses the case with another nurse practitioner. The questions following the case presentation guide the class discussion in areas such as ethics, cultural competency, standards of practice, and overall feelings of the nurse practitioner. Application of this case study can be done in a variety of ways using distance education. To provide the background knowledge on standards of practice, a reading assignment and lecture notes (or podcasted lecture) can be distributed to the online class. A live chat room setting could be used to distribute the case study and then to discuss the case questions. Another discussion method would be to divide the class into teams to discuss the case and then post a summary discussion for the team in the general online classroom. Instructor involvement in the team discussion or in the chat room option would pertain to leading the class to explore different options for providing evidence-based care, solving ethical dilemmas, and investigating cultural norms and competency as well as standards of practice.

EVALUATING THE TECHNOLOGIES USED

Quality Matters (2012) provides basic assessment criteria for the use of technology in online courses. The criteria for course technology are as follows:

- The tools and media support the course learning objectives.
- Course tools and media support student engagement and guide the student to become an active learner.
- Navigation throughout the online components of the course is logical, consistent, and efficient.
- Students can readily access the technologies required in the course.
- The course technologies are current.

Billings and Connors (2012) provide additional criteria for evaluating technology in a distance education course. Nursing programs can use these criteria in a postcourse survey each term.

Access:

- Students can take the course because it is offered on the web.
- Resources for participating in the course are available.

Convenience:

- The course allows students to participate at their own time and pace.
- Synchronous activities (chat, on-campus meetings) are used judiciously.
- Course assignments can be completed conveniently and with resources available at a distance.

Connectedness:

- Students have a sense of being connected to the course and students and faculty in the course.
- There are activities within the course to build connectedness and overcome the isolation that can occur in web courses.

Preparation for real-world work:

- Course activities contribute to the development of the knowledge, skills, and values of the profession.
- Course activities are directed toward application of content in practice settings.

Socialization to the profession:

- Course activities contribute to the development of professional practice roles.
- The course is designed to provide opportunities for students to interact with faculty, preceptors, and others who are able to model professional practice behaviors and the development of professional values.

Satisfaction with web-based learning:

- Students rate the course and instruction positively.
- Students can adapt their learning styles to the strategies of web-based learning.
- Students choose web-based courses as an acceptable or preferred way of learning.

Proficiency with computer skills and use of learning management system tools:

- Students improve in their ability to use the web course tools.
- Students acquire information-seeking and web-based communication skills.

Whichever criteria are chosen for evaluating the use of technology and its influence on assessment of clinical reasoning, critical thinking, or knowledge gain, they need to be measured consistently across courses and across terms. Data collection and presentation of results through faculty meetings and to student groups provide nurse educators with student feedback to improve the educational experience. Just as important are the informal discussions among faculty who share assignments that work well and those that need revision or removal from online courses.

SUMMARY AND KEY POINTS

This chapter covered laying the foundation for design of learning activities, which includes knowing the expected outcomes, knowing the students, assessing available resources, and selecting the right technology. Examples of assignments at different levels of nursing education were provided. With our mandate to transform nursing education, improve clinical reasoning, and bring the bedside into the classroom, technology is an important support to teaching and learning. Creating new and unique assignments, which allow students to demonstrate the course objectives and program outcomes while stimulating their minds, is a worthwhile endeavor for nurse educators.

Key Points

1. Lay the foundation of the course, the choices for assignments, and the use of technology based on the program and course outcomes.
2. Know students by assessing their prior knowledge, level of education, ability to use existing technologies, and limitations such as bandwidth and costs.
3. Assess the available resources provided by book publishers, the campus or university system, and Internet resources that are free or low cost.
4. Select the type of technology that will meet learners' needs and the course outcomes. The type of technology used should support the course objectives, student abilities, and program outcomes.
5. When a design works well, share it with peers. Network with other nursing faculty teaching via distance education and learn what they do well.

6. Evaluate the use of technology in online courses and nursing program by using consistent criteria, such as the criteria provided within the *NLN Living Book*.

REFERENCES

Billings, D. M. & Connors, H. R. (2012). Chapter two. In *NLN Living Book*. Retrieved from http://www.electronicvision.com/nln/chapter02/index.htm

eHow. (2011). How to make a concept map in Microsoft Word. Retrieved from http://www.ehow.com/how_4927645_make-concept-map-microsoft-word.html

Flippin, C. (2010). Case studies: The value of sharing experiences. *Plastic Surgical Nursing, 30*(1), 1–3. Retrieved from http://www.nursingcenter.com/pdf.asp?AID=988645

Hixon, E., Buckenmeyer, J., & Zamojski, H. (2011). Bloom's Taxonomy in a digital age. Retrieved from http://www.uwex.edu/disted/conference/Resource_library/handouts/46402_P.pdf

Jeffries, P. (2011). How to write a case study. Retrieved from http://www.nursingsociety.org/Education/CourseAdoption/Documents/online_howto.pdf

MERLOT Health Sciences Portal. (2012). Teaching health sciences with technology. Retrieved from http://healthsciences.merlot.org/teach.html

Novak, J. D., & Cañas, A. J. (2008). The theory underlying concept maps and how to construct them. Technical report IHMC CmapTools. Retrieved from http://cmap.ihmc.us/Publications/ResearchPapers/TheoryUnderlyingConceptMaps.pdf

Quality Matters. (2012). Rubric standards 2011–2013 edition with assigned point values. Retrieved from http://www.qmprogram.org/files/QM_Standards_20112013.pdf

Rejman, K. (2010). A difficult pregnancy: A nurse practitioner looks for answers. Retrieved from http://sciencecases.lib.buffalo.edu/cs/

Schrock, K. (2011). Bloomin' Google. Google apps to support Bloom's taxonomy. Retrieved from http://kathyschrock.net/googleblooms/

TEN

Enhancing Writing in Online Education

MARILYN H. OERMANN

Learning to communicate ideas in writing is an important outcome of any nursing program and essential for a successful career in nursing. Even though most nurses may not write for publication, they need to express their ideas logically and clearly in documentation, reports, and other written materials. As nurses continue their education, the ability to write scholarly papers, research reports, and clinical papers is critical to their own career development and to nursing as a profession. Development of evidence-based practice depends on nurses disseminating the findings of projects and studies in the clinical setting, which requires written communication skills. Nurses, as leaders in the health system, need to communicate clearly and persuasively in their reports and other documents in the work setting.

The quality of nursing students' writing is often less than desired. Some students enter nursing with limited writing instruction and experience, having completed many objective tests but few scholarly papers. Other factors that can influence writing ability are a lack of understanding of grammar, punctuation, and technical aspects of good writing; English as a second language (ESL); time to think through ideas and the best ways of expressing them; and overuse of informal writing styles seen in e-mail, text messaging, and other forms of Internet communication. Graduate students are at a disadvantage when writing research and clinical papers without a solid foundation in written communication skills at the prelicensure level.

Distance education (DE) programs provide an opportunity to hone and develop excellent writing skills because of the almost daily need to write well-formed, evidence-based discussion responses and assignments. Distance learners often communicate only in writing through discussion question replies, e-mail, instant messaging, chat rooms, and written assignments. Weaknesses in writing skills often become quickly noticeable to the instructor as well as peers.

WRITING ACROSS THE CURRICULUM

Developing the ability to write well is similar to gaining expertise in clinical skills: the learner needs practice combined with feedback and guidance to improve writing. To address the lack of writing skills among students, and provide this needed experience, Writing Across the Curriculum (WAC) programs were developed in the 1980s and continue to be used today. The proponents of WAC programs believe that learning to write is the responsibility of the academic community as a whole, not only the English department, and it requires more than completing an English composition course (WAC Clearinghouse, 2011a). Integration of writing occurs across disciplines with practice in writing incorporated throughout the learner's degree program. The WAC approach is useful for enhancing writing in nursing programs, including DE.

Writing in the Discipline

One important component of WAC programs is learning to write in one's discipline as a means of communicating within the field. Writing to communicate means the student can disseminate ideas understood by readers—the writing informs, explains, directs, and persuades. Writing assignments in a nursing course, such as a paper analyzing a patient's care or a research proposal, introduce students to the language of nursing, and how to communicate to a professional audience, and to new concepts. By writing in the discipline, students learn the writing style and conventions of nursing and its literature, preparing them for eventual membership in the profession (Carter & Rukholm, 2008). Papers in which students consider different perspectives and alternate courses of action encourage higher-level thinking. Writing assignments in nursing can teach students to think like a nurse.

Generally, writing in the discipline includes formal papers that adhere to the format and style of the field (WAC Clearinghouse, 2011b). Examples of this type of assignment in a nursing program are term papers, papers that analyze issues in nursing or argue for a position, literature reviews, systematic reviews, research proposals, and manuscripts written in a nursing course. New electronic methods of communicating nursing trends, issues, policies, opinions, and innovations should be encouraged in DE programs. Assignments such as these teach students how to communicate in the field and enable them to improve and retain their writing ability. Faculty feedback relates to the substance of the document (electronic or paper), the degree to which the student met the criteria of the assignment, the writing style, and overall quality. Thus, with well-designed writing assignments and careful critique and feedback from instructors, students develop skill in writing within the discipline.

The *Essentials of Baccalaureate Education for Professional Nursing Practice* identify the importance of students developing skill in communication, including writing, which is critical to the practice of nursing and the role of the nurse as a professional (American Association of Colleges of Nursing [AACN], 2008). At the master's and doctoral levels, graduates need scholarly writing skills to function as leaders in the health system; disseminate outcomes of clinical projects and innovations; develop and communicate practice guidelines, policies, and standards; and conduct research studies and disseminate their findings (AACN, 2006, 2011). To develop these skills, students need to experience the writing, feedback, and revision process in nursing courses throughout the curriculum.

Writing to Learn

A second component of WAC programs includes writing activities to learn key concepts. The goal is learning, not writing. Writing-to-learn activities, such as listing questions from a reading assignment and recording reflections on clinical practice in a journal, are often short and informal. By keeping these informal, students can think through ideas and question confusing points. For this reason, writing-to-learn activities may be impromptu (WAC Clearinghouse, 2011c). A good example in online classes is asking students to summarize key concepts that are applicable to their practice as nurses at the end of a unit or module. Students could also write questions about key concepts or describe concepts that are confusing to them. Feedback from the teacher on writing-to-learn activities focuses on the content, not on spelling, punctuation, grammar, or writing style. This is in contrast to writing-in-the-discipline assignments that are intended to improve writing ability, with instructor feedback that focuses on writing style and content.

Planning for Writing Assignments

Typically, faculty members plan assignments for their own courses without consideration of writing activities in other courses in the curriculum. Ideally, the curriculum committee or other decision-making group in the nursing program should establish goals for writing across the curriculum. With this approach, formal papers that develop students' ability to write, and require drafts and rewrites, are carefully planned in the curriculum. This approach also considers the time it takes for faculty to provide feedback.

A systematic approach allows faculty to sequence types of papers and other writing assignments through the curriculum in a logical way. For example, to learn about evidence-based practice in a prelicensure nursing program, students might begin by writing a short paper on sources of evidence, followed by an assignment in which they identify a question they have about a patient, search for evidence, and write a summary of their findings. In a later nursing course, students might identify a clinical question, search the literature for relevant studies, critique those studies, and prepare a formal paper. Planning writing assignments through a series of online courses ensures that students will engage in some form of writing in each nursing course to progressively develop their writing skill.

The other advantage of planning writing assignments for the nursing program as a whole is to avoid excessive repetition of assignments (Oermann & Gaberson, 2009). Rather than using the same assignments repetitively in a course or multiple courses, a systematic approach to planning avoids this issue. Writing assignments are not only time consuming for students, but they are also time consuming for faculty.

Purposes of Writing Assignments

Writing assignments in a nursing course, online or face-to-face, are developed based on the outcomes to be met by students. Each assignment in a nursing course should be directly tied to a course objective and carefully planned. Often, long-standing course assignments are no longer the most relevant for the current objectives of the course. Writing assignments, in addition to enhancing students' writing ability, have three main purposes. First, they help students learn about concepts, theories, and other information related to the course outcomes. Second, writing assignments can be used to foster students' critical thinking about a topic and develop their higher-level thinking skills. Third, with writing assignments, students can explore feelings, beliefs, and values.

Journals are one such assignment: students can be guided to reflect on their feelings and experiences and record these in the journal. This reflection on practice is one of the strategies suggested by Benner, Sutphen, Leonard, and Day (2010) to promote formation of inner values associated with professional nursing practice. The format of reflective writing is not critical—it is the substance or level of reflection that is an important element in formation of values (Fischer, Haley, Saarinen, & Chretien, 2011). Blogs for personal reflection and wikis for group formation activities are strategies that can easily be used in online courses.

Formal Papers

Writing assignments to help students improve their writing ability include formal papers, generally completed over time. Table 10.1 provides examples of formal paper assignments in nursing courses. In these papers, students learn how to organize their thoughts and present them clearly. Formal papers provide a means of learning content and improving writing skill, thus allowing nursing faculty to assess both of these areas. Formal papers such as a term paper in a course, research proposal,

TABLE 10.1 Examples of Formal Papers in Nursing Courses

• Term papers related to the objectives of the course
• Papers in which students analyze concepts and theories and their use in clinical practice
• Literature reviews and systematic reviews
• Research proposals and papers
• Papers comparing different interventions with their underlying evidence base
• Critiques and syntheses of evidence
• Critical analysis papers in which students analyze issues, analyze and compare different options, and develop arguments for a position
• Case study analyses with a written rationale and literature to support the analysis
• Papers comparing readings and class content to patient care
• Concept analysis papers in which students describe a concept, its characteristics, and how it applies to care of patients or how it could be used in practice
• Manuscripts

and manuscript provide students an opportunity to use a specific writing style, such as the *Publication Manual of the American Psychological Association* (APA) in their writing (APA, 2010). The focus of these papers is not learning APA style, but rather, thinking about and communicating ideas clearly in written form.

All too often, faculty members focus their assessment and grading on the correct use of APA style in a paper rather than its substance and the quality of the writing. Students often believe that all faculty are looking for is "APA" and not the ideas they spent so much time developing. Giddens and Lobo (2008) had graduate students in a nursing education course grade a mock paper. There was wide variability in scoring and comments, with the majority of comments on APA formatting rather than substantive concerns about the paper. Using a rubric to read and grade the assignments can eliminate some of the focus on writing style by limiting the number of points pertaining to writing style and format. This limit on style and format then refocuses the faculty's grading on the content of the paper.

Writing in the discipline is a competency to be taught by nursing faculty because it is unlikely that students, even those who are good writers, will enter a nursing program knowing how to write clinical and scholarly papers. Beginning nursing courses should introduce students to different forms of nursing literature. Students should read journal articles, the predominant means of keeping up-to-date as a professional, in every nursing course so they become accustomed to searching the literature when they have questions about clinical practice. By reading scholarly, published articles in each nursing course, students can see examples that can serve as a guide for their own writing.

Often, the directions for a paper are not sufficient to guide the writing that is expected. Samples of well-written papers can illustrate effective ways of approaching the writing assignment and what is expected in a "good paper." The teacher can highlight the critical elements demonstrated in the examples. Expectations for written work vary among faculty; thus, preparing the students to meet the expectations is the instructor's responsibility. To improve students' writing ability, nursing faculty in one school of nursing developed an online writing tutorial to teach students to write successfully (Roberts & Goss, 2009). The tutorial included a PowerPoint presentation and video stream on writing style, organizing and presenting ideas, constructing paragraphs and sentences, eliminating common writing errors, conforming to APA style, and referencing ideas. The tutorial also reviewed grammar, punctuation, and other conventions of writing. Students who completed the tutorial showed improvement in their written essays.

As formal papers are completed over time, and nursing students often have competing demands on their time, dividing the paper into smaller segments with specific due dates can help. Smaller, more manageable assignments that build on one another are less daunting for students (Luthy, Peterson, Lassetter, & Callister, 2009). Each of the paper's content areas can represent an individual assignment, with the faculty member providing feedback on those assignments building to the final paper. For example, students might prepare a paper on a quality of care or patient safety issue identified in their practice setting. The first segment of the paper, for review and feedback, might be a description of the issue they observed, including characteristics of the setting and other information they collected related to the issue addressed in the paper. The next segment of the paper might be a literature review on the issue. The third segment of the assignment might be their plan for improvement or how they would address the safety issue in the clinical setting, including interventions to implement, who will be responsible, tests of change to modify the intervention, and an outline for assessing how well the intervention was implemented and for evaluating its effectiveness.

With careful planning, formal papers in a course can be integrated with other types of learning activities. For example, a series of well-crafted discussion questions can also lead the student through writing the final formal paper or project for a course while receiving instructor and peer feedback throughout the entire online course. The sharing of ideas in the discussions can expand all students' knowledge and beliefs on the topic. The faculty member's intentional feedback and discussion responses can promote writing and thinking skills within the course.

Learning to Write Formal Papers

Writing a paper requires planning, organization, and personal strategies to pace writing. Prewriting activities allow students to focus on their writing once they begin and not be distracted by other tasks (Oermann & Hays, 2011). Preparing an outline and keeping supporting documents (journal articles, texts) nearby are beginning steps nursing students may not know about. Outlines allow students to plan content areas, order them logically, and ensure that the requirements of the paper will be met. For formal papers, the content areas listed in the outline can then be used as headings and subheadings in the paper (Oermann & Hays, 2011).

Drafts, in most instances, are used as a means of providing feedback to students and are not graded. In writing the first draft, students should write quickly to get their ideas on paper (Oermann, 2010; Oermann & Hays, 2011). Once the content is adequate, grammar, spelling, punctuation, and writing style can be revised. Although time consuming for faculty, having an opportunity to get feedback on writing and being able to rewrite based on those suggestions is valuable in improving writing ability.

Writing-to-Learn Activities

Writing-to-learn activities are often impromptu. In contrast to formal papers, writing-to-learn activities engage students in learning and thinking about the topic but are not intended to improve writing as a skill. An online class might begin with students writing one question they had from their reading assignment or prior class, or they might be asked to respond to a writing prompt about their clinical experience, for example, what did you learn today in clinical practice that will be of value in your future practice? After reading a series of comments in a discussion board, the teacher may identify a gap in learning and ask students to respond to questions about the key concepts they should have learned in class or through their readings. Students might exchange responses with each other to confirm they understand the content. Table 10.2 provides some examples of writing-to-learn activities in nursing courses.

ASSESSMENT OF WRITING ASSIGNMENTS

Assessment involves reviewing the paper and providing feedback to students that guides subsequent revision of the assignment or future assignments. Teachers should assess papers for accuracy and comprehensiveness of the content, organization, choice of words, and effectiveness in conveying ideas. They also should assess writing style and technique such as paragraph and sentence structure, punctuation, grammar, spelling, accuracy, and format of the references (Oermann & Gaberson, 2009; Oermann & Hays, 2011).

Providing Feedback

Feedback that is prompt, specific, and instructional is critical for learning. The goal of feedback is not to rewrite the entire paper for the

TABLE 10.2 Examples of Writing-to-Learn Activities in Nursing Courses

• Responses to writing prompts
• Developing and answering questions about an online class or readings
• Summaries of readings
• Annotated bibliographies
• Journals and reflective writing activities
• Short clinical papers
• Analyses of clinical scenarios
• Case studies
• Nursing care plans
• Teaching plans
• Concept maps with rationale
• Write-ups of assessments, physical examinations
• Analyses of interactions with individuals and groups
• Process analyses (describing in writing the steps required to complete a process)

student. As a strategy to avoid this tendency, the teacher can indicate writing errors with highlighting (or inserting comments in an electronic document), include notes that explain the errors, and require students to rewrite those sections in a subsequent draft or for the teacher to check. For example, rather than indicating that "content is not well organized," more effective feedback would be that "the data on the patient's prior health problems and family's responses should be presented together rather than having this scattered throughout pages 3 to 7." In some cases, the faculty member may go one step further to correct selected writing errors for students. However, this should be done only if the teacher believes that demonstrating the revisions would be valuable to guide student development.

Luthy and colleagues (2009) suggested that students be required to have their papers reviewed first by peers to improve the quality of the paper before submitting to the faculty member. As feedback is time consuming, the teacher can have students critique each other's writing in pairs or in small groups with online tools. Peers can provide feedback on the accuracy of the content, its organization, and the clarity of writing. Peers may not notice errors in grammar and punctuation, but generally, they can determine if the paper does not communicate ideas clearly. When peer assessment is used, the faculty member should specify guidelines for the critique.

A wiki is a web-based program in which students can work collaboratively on a document in real time (Collier, 2010). Students post their papers, or sections of it, on the wiki, and peers and the instructor provide feedback for revising the papers. Wikispaces (www.wikispaces.com) is a free service faculty might use for team projects or individual projects in which classmates add to a writing assignment. Another strategy is for students to post writing questions for faculty and peers in an online discussion board (McMillan & Raines, 2010).

Grading Writing Assignments

Summative evaluation of completed writing assignments is intended for grading. Criteria for assessing the quality of formal papers and other writing assignments are presented in Table 10.3. Using these criteria, the teacher can develop a scoring rubric to guide grading of the assignment. A rubric lists the criteria to be met or areas to be included in the paper with the allotted points (Oermann & Gaberson, 2009). Some instructors include the writing assignment instructions and outline within the grading rubric. Doing so makes it clear what is to be included in the assignment and how each section is graded.

There are two types of rubrics for grading writing assignments. A holistic rubric lists the areas of the paper to be considered in the evaluation, but the teacher grades the paper as a whole without scoring each individual area (Table 10.4). The holistic rubric lacks specificity in determining the points for the grade. In contrast, an analytic rubric lists each individual area of a paper to be assessed with the points allotted for that area. The grade for the assignment is the total score (Table 10.5).

Other Principles for Assessing Writing Assignments

If graded, writing assignments should be read anonymously to avoid bias. The teacher may have a general impression of the student, which can inadvertently influence the assessment and scoring. To improve the grading of formal papers, Bickes and Schim (2010) recommend a system of blind review by instructors who are not involved in teaching the students. In their course, students submit the drafts to their clinical instructors for feedback, but the final paper is given to the course coordinator, who removes identifying information and assigns a code number to each paper. The final papers are graded by a different faculty member than the

TABLE 10.3 Criteria for Assessing Papers and Other Writing Assignments

Content
- Content is relevant.
- Content is accurate.
- Significant concepts and theories are presented.
- Concepts and theories are used appropriately for analysis.
- Content is comprehensive.
- Content reflects current research.
- Hypotheses, conclusions, and decisions are supported.

Organization
- Content is organized logically.
- Ideas are presented in logical sequence.
- Paragraph structure is appropriate.
- Headings are used appropriately to indicate new content areas.

Process
- Process used to arrive at solutions, approaches, decisions, and so forth is adequate.
- Consequences of decisions are considered and weighed.
- Sound rationale is provided based on theory and research as appropriate.
- For papers analyzing issues, rationale supports position taken.
- Multiple perspectives and new approaches are considered.

Writing style
- Ideas are described clearly.
- Sentence structure is clear.
- There are no grammatical errors.
- There are no spelling errors.
- Appropriate punctuation is used.
- Writing does not reveal bias related to gender, sexual orientation, racial or ethnic identity, or disabilities.
- Length of paper is consistent with requirements.
- References are cited appropriately throughout paper.
- References are cited accurately according to required format.

Reprinted with permission from Gaberson and Oermann (2010, p. 363).

student had in clinical practice, removing the potential for personal bias in the grading process.

Oermann and Gaberson (2009) suggested that another reason to grade papers anonymously is to prevent a carryover effect, in which the teacher recalls and carries over from prior assignments to the current one an assumption about the quality of the student's writing. If the student scored low on one paper, the teacher may expect the next paper to also be poorly done and written. When assessing multiple parts of a writing assignment, prior parts that were scored should be covered up to avoid this potential problem in the evaluation. Also, student papers should be read in random order. Papers read early may receive higher scores than those read near the end because of teacher fatigue and time constraints (Oermann & Gaberson, 2009). This also means that faculty

TABLE 10.4 Sample Holistic Scoring Rubric for Formal Papers and Other Writing Assignments

Score of 3
- Content is accurate, relevant to goals of paper, complete, in depth
- Research findings and other evidence support ideas in paper
- Relevant literature cited
- Purpose of paper stated clearly
- Content well organized and flows logically
- Thorough discussion of ideas with multiple perspectives considered
- Effective conclusions with implications
- Paragraphs appropriate; sentence structure clear; no errors in grammar, punctuation, or spelling
- Paper meets all requirements of assignment
- Appropriate references, no errors in APA style

Score of 2
- Most content accurate, content relevant to goals of paper but lacks depth
- Relevant research and evidence cited
- Relevant literature used but not in depth
- Purpose stated but not well developed
- Content organized logically
- Adequate discussion of ideas with some alternate perspectives
- Adequate summary of main ideas but limited implications
- Paragraphs adequate; sentence structure and transitions adequate; some grammar, punctuation, and spelling errors
- Some elements of paper missing or too short
- References relevant but limited, most current; some errors in APA style

Score of 1
- Some content not accurate, some content not relevant to goals of paper, content lacks depth
- Limited research and evidence cited in paper
- Limited literature used to support ideas
- Purpose poorly developed, not stated clearly
- Content poorly organized
- Ideas not developed adequately, discussion lacks detail and is incomplete, no alternate perspectives mentioned
- Poor conclusion, no synthesis, no implications
- Paragraphs not developed adequately; poor sentence structure and transitions; many errors in grammar, punctuation, and spelling
- Missing parts of paper
- Few references, many old; errors in references and APA style

should plan for time to read student work when fatigue and time constraints are less.

Formal papers and other writing assignments should be read twice before scoring. In the first reading, the teacher can suggest revisions and add comments about the content, organization of the paper, and writing. By reading all the papers first, comparing them to the grading rubric but not yet scoring the assignment, the teacher may find that none of the

TABLE 10.5 Sample Analytic Scoring Rubric for Formal Papers and Other Writing Assignments

Content		
Content relevant to purpose of paper, comprehensive and in depth	Content relevant to purpose of paper	Some content not relevant to purpose of paper, lacks depth
10 9 8	7 6 5 4	3 2 1
Content accurate	Most of content accurate	Major errors in content
10 9 8	7 6 5 4	3 2 1
Sound background developed from concepts, theories, and literature	Background relevant to topic but limited development	Background not developed, limited support for ideas
20–15	14–7	6–1
Current research synthesized and integrated effectively in paper	Relevant research summarized in paper	Limited research in paper, not used to support ideas
10 9 8	7 6 5 4	3 2 1
Organization		
Purpose of paper/thesis well developed and clearly stated	Purpose/thesis apparent but not developed sufficiently	Purpose/thesis poorly developed, not clear
5	4 3 2	1
Ideas well organized and logically presented, organization supports arguments and development of ideas	Clear organization of main points and ideas	Poorly organized, ideas not developed adequately in paper
10 9 8	7 6 5 4	3 2 1
Thorough discussion of ideas, includes multiple perspectives and new approaches	Adequate discussion of ideas, some alternate perspectives considered	Discussion not thorough, lacks detail, no alternate perspectives considered
10 9 8	7 6 5 4	3 2 1
Effective conclusion and integration of ideas in summary	Adequate conclusion, summary of main ideas	Poor conclusion, no integration of ideas
5	4 3 2	1

(*continued*)

TABLE 10.5 Sample Analytic Scoring Rubric for Formal Papers and Other Writing Assignments (continued)

	Writing style and format	
Sentence structure clear, smooth transitions, correct grammar and punctuation, no spelling errors	Adequate sentence structure and transitions; few grammar, punctuation, and spelling errors	Poor sentence structure and transitions; errors in grammar, punctuation, and spelling
10 9 8	7 6 5 4	3 2 1
Professional appearance of paper, all parts included, length consistent with requirements	Paper legible, some parts missing or too short/too long considering requirements	Unprofessional appearance, missing sections, paper too short/too long considering requirements
5	4 3 2	1
References used appropriately in paper, references current, no errors in references, correct use of APA style for references	References used appropriately in paper but limited, most references current, some citations or references with errors and/or some errors in APA style for references	Few references and limited breadth, old references (not classic), errors in references, errors in APA style for references
5	4 3 2	1
Total points _______ (sum points for total score)		

Reprinted with permission from Oermann and Gaberson (2009, pp. 237–238).

students addressed certain content areas. With this approach, the teacher can modify the criteria and rubric and easily change the comments made on the electronic version of the paper (Oermann & Gaberson, 2009). The second reading of the assignment is for the actual scoring of the paper and final feedback. In online courses, feedback on papers is best provided electronically using tools such as Microsoft® Word's track changes and insertion of comments.

PREVENTING PLAGIARISM

There are many ethical issues that students need to learn about when communicating their ideas in writing. They need to be accurate in using references, both in how they present the ideas of others and the actual citations. Students need to understand copyright, preventing them from copying the work of others and using it in their own papers without citing the original source. They cannot use text, tables, figures, and other graphics in their papers without permission and cannot use text from websites without referencing the original source. Kenny (2007) suggested that the availability of the Internet and its many resources has led to an increase in nursing students plagiarizing in their papers.

The first step in preventing plagiarism is to ensure students understand what it is, what is acceptable behavior when it comes to writing, and how to acknowledge sources of information. They should know how to paraphrase, summarize, and quote. Reading a statement in the syllabus and engaging in an online discussion about plagiarism are not the same as translating that information into one's own writing. For many learners, plagiarism is a vague concept, and for this reason, it is valuable to provide examples of plagiarism for students to analyze and discuss. The teacher can develop a learning activity in which students read an article or a section of a chapter and a sample paper written using that source. The task for students is to identify instances of plagiarism in the sample text and explain why, check the use of citations, and correct the text. Writing-to-learn activities can be developed in which students read a short passage and paraphrase the text, comparing what they wrote to the original source. Peers also can review each other's writing to confirm proper practices. Other strategies proposed earlier for formal papers, such as dividing papers into smaller segments for review and feedback with deadlines for submission, prevent students from attempting to write their papers at the last minute and may minimize pressure to plagiarize.

Some students are well aware that they are plagiarizing in their papers. They may be pressured to do well on an assignment, be unprepared for the writing, or lack the time and skills to write the paper (Fischer & Zigmond, 2011). For these reasons and others, students may be pressured to copy and paste text from an article, a website, or a friend's paper. In other words, they plagiarize intentionally. More likely, though, the student's plagiarism is unintentional. Many nursing students have not had experiences that prepare them to write a scholarly paper, including reviewing the literature and citing sources as support. Students with English as a second language may not only lack the experience but also may not understand when and how to cite others' ideas in a paper. ESL students may not have sufficient vocabulary to paraphrase.

Students should be told explicitly to avoid copying and pasting from an original source or writing with the intention of later adding the citations. Over time, it is easy to forget that they did not write the material themselves and where references are needed. This is a hazard particularly for research and other formal papers prepared over a period of weeks or longer. Students should insert the references as they are writing the first draft, without concern about the citation format. This is easy to do with bibliographic management software, but even without such software, they can type the references in parentheses as they are drafting the text.

Bristol (2011) proposed three components to preventing plagiarism: having a policy that clearly defines plagiarism, consistent with the policies of the nursing department and college; preparing faculty and students in using plagiarism-detection tools and resources; and using individualized strategies to help students understand plagiarism and how to avoid it in their own writing. The policy should be in the syllabus and should outline consequences of plagiarism. Bristol also recommended that schools of nursing have policies on the use of plagiarism-detecting software, whether faculty or students submit the assignments, types of written assignments, and the acceptable level of originality.

In a study of the impact of plagiarism-detecting software programs in accounting, writing assignments of 338 students were analyzed. Plagiarism decreased by 77% when plagiarism detection software was used in addition to strict academic penalties for students who plagiarized assignments (Tackett, Claypool, Wolf, & Antenucci, 2010). In another study, students were informed that their papers would be put through plagiarism detection software, and they would be penalized if they were found to plagiarize. Students plagiarized significantly less than prior groups of students ($p < .001$; Bilic-Zulle, Azman, Frkovic, & Petrovecki, 2008). There are many plagiarism detecting software programs available, and faculty should evaluate products before selecting them for use in their courses. Students should know at the outset that this software will be used. Students can submit their own papers to these programs before submitting them for a grade, which may decrease the incidence of plagiarism.

SUMMARY AND KEY POINTS

Writing assignments in online courses that prepare students to communicate effectively are critical for their future role as nursing professionals. The WAC approach is useful as a framework for planning writing assignments in nursing programs. It includes learning to write in one's discipline as a means of communicating within the field and writing-to-learn activities.

Ideally, writing assignments are carefully integrated in the curriculum, allowing students to write across a course or series of online courses while receiving feedback. Feedback should be prompt, specific, and informative. The criteria for evaluation of papers and any rubric used to guide grading should relate to the outcomes of the assignment, be used consistently for scoring all of the papers, and be reviewed with learners before they start to write. The ability to write well is as important as other skills we teach in nursing programs. It is a responsibility of the nurse educator to teach students what good writing is and provide constructive and specific feedback for improvement.

Key Points

1. DE learners often communicate only in writing, and DE courses provide outstanding opportunities to improve writing skills.
2. The four main purposes of writing assignments are to enhance writing ability; help students learn about concepts, theories, and other information; foster students' critical thinking about a topic and develop higher-level thinking skills; and explore feelings, beliefs, and values.
3. Writing assignments within the DE classroom include formal papers, writing-to-learn activities, discussion questions, chat rooms and blogs, and team discussion groups.
4. Feedback is critical for students and should be prompt, specific, and instructional.
5. Three suggested components to prevent plagiarism are to have a policy that clearly defines plagiarism, prepare faculty and students in using plagiarism detection tools and resources, and use individualized strategies to help students understand plagiarism and how to avoid it in their own writing.

REFERENCES

American Association of Colleges of Nursing (AACN). (2006). *The essentials of doctoral education for advanced nursing practice*. Washington, DC: AACN.

AACN. (2008). *The essentials of baccalaureate education for professional nursing practice*. Washington, DC: AACN.

AACN. (2011). *The essentials of master's education in nursing*. Washington, DC: AACN.

American Psychological Association (APA). (2010). *Publication manual of the American Psychological Association* (6th ed.). Washington, DC: Author.

Benner, P., Sutphen, M., Leonard, V., & Day, L. (2010). *Educating nurses: A call for radical transformation*. San Francisco: Jossey-Bass. Retrieved from http://www.carnegiefoundation.org/publications/educating-nurses-call-radical-transformation

Bickes, J. T., & Schim, S. M. (2010). Righting writing: Strategies for improving nursing student papers. *International Journal of Nursing Education Scholarship*, 7(1), Art. 8. doi:10.2202/1548-923X.1964

Bilic-Zulle, L., Azman, J., Frkovic, V., & Petrovecki, M. (2008). Is there an effective approach to deterring students from plagiarizing? *Science and Engineering Ethics, 14,* 139–147.

Bristol, T. J. (2011). Plagiarism prevention with technology. *Teaching & Learning in Nursing, 6,* 146–149.

Carter, L. M., & Rukholm, E. (2008). A study of critical thinking, teacher–student interaction, and discipline-specific writing in an online educational setting for registered nurses. *Journal of Continuing Education in Nursing, 39,* 133–138.

Collier, J. (2010). Wiki technology in the classroom: Building collaboration skills. *Journal of Nursing Education, 49,* 718.

Fischer, B. A., & Zigmond, M. J. (2011). Educational approaches for discouraging plagiarism. *Urologic Oncology: Seminars and Original Investigations, 29,* 100–103.

Fischer, M. A., Haley, H., Saarinen, C. L., & Chretien, K. C. (2011). Comparison of blogged and written reflections in two medicine clerkships. *Medical Education, 45,* 166–175.

Gaberson, K., & Oermann, M. H. (2010). *Clinical teaching strategies in nursing* (3rd ed.). New York, NY: Springer Publishing.

Giddens, J. F., & Lobo, M. (2008). Analyzing graduate student trends in written paper evaluation. *Journal of Nursing Education, 47,* 480–483.

Kenny, D. (2007). Student plagiarism and professional practice. *Nurse Education Today, 27*(1), 14–18.

Luthy, K. E., Peterson, N. E., Lassetter, J. H., & Callister, L. C. (2009). Successfully incorporating Writing Across the Curriculum with advanced writing in nursing. *Journal of Nursing Education, 48,* 54–59.

McMillan, L., & Raines, K. (2010). Headed in the "write" direction: Nursing student publication and health promotion in the community. *Journal of Nursing Education, 49,* 418–421.

Oermann, M. H. (2010). Writing for publication in nursing: What every nurse educator needs to know. In L. Caputi (Ed.), *Teaching nursing: The art and science* (2nd ed., pp. 146–166). Glen Ellyn, IL: College of DuPage.

Oermann, M. H., & Gaberson, K. B. (2009). *Evaluation and testing in nursing education* (3rd ed.). New York, NY: Springer Publishing.

Oermann, M. H., & Hays, J. (2011). *Writing for publication in nursing* (2nd ed.). New York, NY: Springer Publishing.

Roberts, S. T., & Goss, G. (2009). Use of an online writing tutorial to improve writing skills in nursing courses. *Nurse Educator, 34,* 262–265.

Tackett, J., Claypool, G. A., Wolf, F., & Antenucci, J. (2010). The impact of plagiarism detection software on college plagiarism. *Journal of Business and Accounting, 3,* 68–80.

WAC Clearinghouse. (2011a). *Basic principles of WAC.* Retrieved from http://wac.colostate.edu/intro/pop3a.cfm

WAC Clearinghouse. (2011b). *What is writing in the disciplines?* Retrieved from http://wac.colostate.edu/intro/pop2e.cfm

WAC Clearinghouse. (2011c). *What is writing to learn?* Retrieved from http://wac.colostate.edu/intro/pop2d.cfm

ELEVEN

Quality Monitoring and Accreditation in Nursing Distance Education Programs

DIANE M. BILLINGS, SUZANNE S. DICKERSON, MARY J. GREENBERG, BILL WU YOW-WU, and BRENDA S. TALLEY

Nursing faculty and students have been using distance education (DE) technologies to establish access to academic and continuing-education programs for several decades. The popularity of distance accessible education has increased recently as schools of nursing reform academic programs to meet recommendations from reports such as the Institute of Medicine (IOM) report, *The Future of Nursing*, to have a better-prepared nursing workforce, resulting in a growth of RN-BSN and doctoral programs (both DNP and PhD) being delivered in online or blended formats. Although previous controversy about the effectiveness of distance accessible programs has abated, there is a continued need to monitor quality of nursing courses and programs and ensure that accreditation standards and quality indicators are being met. The purposes of this chapter are to provide a background on quality monitoring (QM) in nursing education, identify current quality indicators for DE, describe a process for QM for evidence-based decision making, describe frameworks for QM, and describe regulations and accreditation standards that pertain to DE in nursing education. The chapter concludes with an exemplar of QM in a PhD program.

QM: EVIDENCE FOR BEST PRACTICES FOR DE IN NURSING

Since the use of DE in nursing education first became popular in the late 1980s and 1990s, nurse educators have conducted a variety of studies to determine evidence of quality in DE programs. Early studies focused on student satisfaction, convenience of DE, issues related to student support, student (and faculty) isolation, and problems with technology and technology support (Billings, 2007). As the technology and teaching–learning practices improved, the foci of QM have shifted to a better understanding of the roles of faculty and students, how to create online communities of professional practice, which type of learners and learning styles are most effective, how to prepare graduates for professional roles, strategies to promote retention and prevent attrition, and how to blend the best of on-campus learning and DE. By using testable models, and valid and reliable instruments, findings from these studies provide a foundation for understanding and evolving the best practices in DE.

Effectiveness of DE Delivery

There have been innumerable studies on the effectiveness of DE in nursing, and virtually all studies reveal few or no significant differences when comparing DE courses with on-campus or blended courses. Early studies used course grades as the measure of learning outcomes, and regardless of the type of technology used, students learned (Billings & Bachmeier, 1994). More recent studies on online courses reveal that student achievement is similar in online courses and in the classroom (Bata-Jones & Avery, 2004; Leasure, Davis, & Thievon, 2000; Lerners, Wilson, & Sitzman, 2007; Little, 2009; Mancuso-Murphy, 2007). Coose (2010) compared students in an ASN program who participated in the program on campus with those who used distance delivery methods and found no differences between students' perception of the effectiveness of the two programs, and there were no differences in learning achievement. In another study, Buckley (2003) reported that there were no differences in learning outcomes among a classroom, a web-enhanced, and a web-based nutrition course for undergraduate nursing students. In general, comparative media studies such as those reported here typically reveal no significant differences in learning outcomes; thus, nurse educators can be assured that offering courses using a variety of DE delivery mechanisms will not compromise learning outcomes.

Use of Teaching–Learning Practices

DE changes classroom dynamics from an emphasis on teaching to a focus on the learner and learning. The role of the faculty is to establish a learning environment that encourages students to explore and solve clinical problems. Faculty are content experts and instructional planners as they work with other experts such as instructional designers, graphic artists, web programmers, and multimedia developers to develop modules, courses, and programs and to select appropriate teaching methods and evaluation. The role of the learner also changes from passive recipient to active knowledge seeker as students assume responsibility for their own learning. Students learn more effectively when they are actively involved, cognitively and socially engaged, and interacting with the content and class members. The course must be designed from the outset to create activities that require active learning (Phillips, 2005).

Learning improves and is shaped by feedback from faculty, peers, preceptors, and mentors. Feedback is most helpful when it occurs in a timely manner and provides information about progress as well as process (Bonnel, 2008). Bonnel recommends designing courses and learning activities to increase the opportunities for students to receive feedback and engage in self-reflection about their learning. Learning is enhanced by engagement and interaction by faculty and classmates with others in the course and by a sense of social presence. Mayne and Wu (2011) found that when intentionally adding strategies to promote social presence and group interaction, students perceived that their expectations for online learning were met. Cobb, Billings, Mays, and Canty-Mitchell (2001) reported a strong relationship among social presence, satisfaction, and instructor performance. Broome, Halstead, Pesut, Rawl, and Boland (2011) found that the sense of isolation in DE programs can be reduced by admitting students in cohorts, having on-campus orientation and socialization sessions, and using technology to support synchronous learning using audio and video. Learning is promoted by meaningful interactions with faculty both inside and outside the course. In DE, both students and faculty must strive to overcome the isolation imposed by distance in order to create opportunities for interaction.

DE and Clinical Practice

Studies on course quality can also be conducted when the course is a clinical course or a didactic course with a clinical component. Lashley (2005) found that in a physical assessment course, students did learn the clinical skills and clinical decision-making outcomes for the course. Faculty used e-mail and chat as well as discussion forums to link students to their instructors, classmates, preceptors, expert nurses, health care professionals, and clients in the broader community of professional practice. Online components of the course can also be used for debriefing actual and simulated clinical experiences. Pullen (2006) found that online learning, when used for continuing professional development, increased learning and knowledge outcomes and resulted in improvement in clinical practice. Nesler, Hanner, Melburg, and McGowan (2001) reported that working with preceptors was a way to foster professional role development.

Student Satisfaction

Student satisfaction continues to be a major element of QM. Student satisfaction with the experience of DE is important to faculty, educational providers, and the students themselves. When compared to similar educational experiences in the on-campus classroom, many students report general levels of satisfaction and indicate they would take DE courses again. Satisfaction is likely related to expectations of how the course will meet learner needs and is dependent on prepared faculty and functioning course-delivery technology. DeBourgh (2003) found that student satisfaction with computer-mediated DE is most associated with the perceived quality of the instruction and the effectiveness of the instructor. Ali, Hodson-Carlton, and Ryan (2004) found that graduate nursing students were satisfied with the flexibility and convenience of online learning and that timely feedback from faculty was a very important indicator of student satisfaction. Doctoral students in a study conducted by Lerners, Wilson, and Sitzman (2007) reported satisfaction with the access to the doctoral program and the ability to enroll in a doctoral program while continuing their employment. In their PhD program, Broome et al. (2011) found that 94% of students were satisfied with the distance accessible program.

Professional Practice Socialization

Nursing is a clinical practice profession, and roles are developed through mentoring, working with expert nurses, and establishing collegial peer groups and networks. Although DE has the potential to isolate learners from faculty, peers, and role models, and thus decrease socialization opportunities, the research tends to show otherwise when specific strategies, such as chat rooms, webinars/web conferencing, and peer mentors, are used to overcome the barriers of distance. Lerners, Wilson, and

Sitzman (2007) found that students believed they were being prepared for professional practice and because of mentoring in the online course, were becoming socialized. Similarly, Broome et al. (2011) described the importance of mentoring in a PhD program to promote socialization to the role of scholar.

Access and Enrollment

Likely underreported is the impact of increased enrollment in academic programs because of the access and convenience of making courses and programs distance accessible. Effken (2008) noted an increase in the pool of potential students in her distance accessible PhD program, and Broome et al. (2011) reported an increase in applicants once the PhD program was available at a distance.

Student Orientation for Technology Use

Students must be oriented to use technology. This can be accomplished by using student handbooks, posting orientation information on the Internet, conducting orientation sessions on campus or at the outreach site prior to the use of the technology, or using the technology itself during the first class session. Carruth, Broussard, Waldmeier, Gauthier, and Mixon (2010) developed a 5-day orientation program for their graduate students to ensure they were prepared to participate in their online course.

Learning Resources and Student Support Services

Learning resources and student services sufficient to support the course must be available for students who are at a distance from the originating site of the educational offering. For example, academic advising, access to the bookstore, registration, bursar, and financial aid services all have to be available to students without their coming to campus. Additional services include learning assessment, career development, learning portfolio management, and competency testing. Of key importance is access to library materials, which typically can be accessed online or be made available at outreach learning centers or by using course pack preparation services that obtain copyright permission for required course readings.

Faculty Development and Workload

Teaching, particularly in online courses, changes the focus from an emphasis on teaching to an emphasis on learning, and because learning occurs through interaction with faculty, peers, and preceptors, learner-centered, constructivist, and sociocultural models provide theoretical guidance for selecting learning activities. Making these shifts requires extensive changes to the design of learning activities (Zsohar & Smith, 2008). Overall, online courses have been found to be more time consuming than traditional classroom teaching (Effken, 2008). Faculty workload increases in DE courses because of the time needed for orientation to the technology and to develop new teaching materials, learning activities, and evaluation strategies. Ali et al. (2004) reported an increase in time spent developing and teaching an online course. Anderson and Avery (2008) found that the time teaching an online course was similar to that teaching an on-campus course, but the preparation time was greater for developing the online course. Developing courses for DE is increasingly becoming dependent on a team of technical and pedagogical experts. Faculty need assistance with designing instructional material, using new teaching methods appropriate to the DE delivery system, and using evaluation strategies that can be implemented within the limits of the DE technology. Broome et al. (2011) recommend workload release or credit during development of DE courses.

QUALITY INDICATORS FOR DISTANCE DELIVERED ACADEMIC PROGRAMS AND COURSES

DE is a complex and dynamic interaction among the use of technology, teaching–learning practices, and the outcomes of distance accessible courses and programs. In order to ensure quality and to guide quality-monitoring efforts, several organizations have developed quality indicators or benchmarks for monitoring quality in an entire program or in a specific course or set of courses.

Monitoring Quality in Academic Programs and Courses

In response to the growing number of universities and for-profit schools that are offering complete degree programs, national groups have developed indicators of good practice for DE programs and evaluation of courses. These guidelines can be used with other campus- or profession-specific guidelines and accreditation criteria. The groups are the Western Interstate Commission for Higher Education (WICHE) and Sloan-C. WICHE developed a set of guidelines to ensure quality in courses developed for adults and offered at a distance (WICHE, 2011). Table 11.1 includes the guidelines listed in *The Principles of Good Practice for Higher Education Institutions Serving Adults at a Distance.*

Sloan-C

The Sloan Consortium also developed quality indicators for use at institutions with distance delivered programs. Based on the premise that learning online should be at least as effective as learning in other modes, Sloan-C offers five pillars of essential elements of quality in an online program (Moore, 2011). These pillars include learning effectiveness, cost effectiveness and institutional commitment, access, faculty satisfaction, and student satisfaction. The framework for Sloan-C can be found in Table 11.2 and at sloanconsortium.org/5pillars.

Evaluating the effectiveness of the teaching and learning that occurs at the course level is equally important and occurs concurrently with monitoring the overall quality of the academic program. Monitoring course quality assumes additional significance when only one or several courses of the entire academic program are offered in a distance-accessible format. While nurse educators are accustomed to conducting evaluations of courses, teaching practices, and learning outcomes, the process and indicators for monitoring these elements require modification for DE offerings. Several frameworks have been developed for QM in courses.

Seven Principles for Good Practice in Undergraduate Education

The Seven Principles for Good Practice in Undergraduate Education (Chickering & Gamson, 1987) have been used as indicators of the quality of teaching and learning in DE courses. These principles include active learning, time on task, collaboration with peers, interaction with faculty, rich and rapid feedback, high expectations, and respect for diversity; these principles also are enabled by DE technologies (Chickering & Ehrmann, 1996). These principles, when applied consistently, result in student learning and satisfaction (Billings, Connors, & Skiba, 2001; Broome et al., 2011). The principles of good practices in education serve as organizing variables for the educational-practices component of the framework for assessing the teaching and learning practices that are used in DE courses.

TABLE 11.1 WICHE Principles of Good Practice (2011)

Criteria	Description
Mission, goals, and objectives	Distance education programs are consistent with the institution's mission and goals, and distance education is an integral component of the institution's mission.
Accountability to stakeholders	To meet this principle, the institution demonstrates its accountability by sharing data about outcomes and results of program reviews and accreditation.
Responsiveness	The institution is responsive to adult learners and develops programs to meet their needs.
Curriculum development and revision	The curriculum is developed based on academic program guidelines and using good practices in design of distance education. The curriculum is reviewed and revised periodically.
Curriculum delivery	The programs and courses are comparable regardless of the delivery method; distance delivered courses are of the same quality as those offered on campus.
Interaction and student engagement	The program and courses are designed to foster interaction between the student and faculty and among and between students.
Faculty qualifications and training	Faculty meet qualifications for teaching in the program as defined by the accrediting bodies and requirements for appointment at the institution. There is appropriate orientation and support for faculty who teach at a distance, including use of technology and teaching and learning strategies.
Faculty evaluation	There are policies in place to evaluate faculty performance.
Student evaluation	Student performance is measured in a timely manner; grading polices are public, and policies are in place about withdrawal, incomplete grades, and academic progression.
Learning outcomes assessment	There is a systematic process for evaluating learning outcomes; results are used for course and program improvement.
Institutional integrity	The institution is regionally accredited and maintains responsibility for outsourced work.
Disclosure	Marketing and communications are accurate and truthful. Information such as recruitment processes, tuition, fees, and course transfer policies are disclosed.
Services	There are sufficient academic and administrative services to support students and faculty.
Resources	There are sufficient resources to ensure a quality educational experience.
Institutional outcomes	Outcomes are measured and published.

Adapted from WICHE (2011).

TABLE 11.2 Sloan-C Quality Framework

	Pillar 1: Learning Effectiveness
Goal	The quality of learning online is demonstrated to be at least as good as the institutional norm.
Process/practice	Academic integrity and control reside with faculty in the same way as in traditional programs at the provider institution.
Metric	Faculty perception surveys or sampled interviews compare learning effectiveness in delivery modes. Learner/graduate/employer focus groups or interviews measure learning gains.
Progress indices	Faculty report that online learning is equivalent or better. Direct assessment of student learning is equivalent or better.
	Pillar 2: Cost Effectiveness and Institutional Commitment
Goal	The institution continuously improves services while reducing costs.
Process/practice	The institution demonstrates financial and technical commitment to its online programs. Tuition rates provide a fair return to the institution and best value to learners.
Metric	Institutional stakeholders show support for participation in online education. Effective practices are identified and shared.
Progress indices	The institution sustains the program, expands and scales upward as desired, and strengthens and disseminates its mission.
	Effective practices and core values are identified and shared through online education. Program entry and support processes inform learners of opportunities and ensure that qualified, motivated learners have reliable access.
	Pillar 3: Access
Goal	All learners who wish to learn online can access learning in a wide array of programs and courses.
Process/practice	Program entry and support processes inform learners of opportunities and ensure that qualified, motivated learners have reliable access.
Metric	Administrative and technical infrastructure provides access to all prospective and enrolled learners. Quality metrics are available for information dissemination, learning resource delivery, and tutoring services.
Progress indices	Qualitative indicators show continuous improvement in growth and effectiveness rates
	Pillar 4: Faculty Satisfaction
Goal	Faculty are pleased with teaching online, citing appreciation and happiness.

(*continued*)

TABLE 11.2 Sloan-C Quality Framework (continued)

Process/practice	Processes ensure faculty participation and support in online education (e.g., governance, intellectual property, royalty sharing, training, preparation, rewards, incentives, and so on).
Metric	Repeat teaching of online courses by individual faculty members indicates approval. Addition of new faculty members shows growing endorsement.
Progress indices	Data from postcourse surveys show continuous improvement. At least 90% of faculty believe that the overall online teaching/learning experience is positive. Willingness/desire to teach additional courses in the program is 80% positive.
	Pillar 5: Student Satisfaction
Goal	Students are pleased with their experiences in learning online, including interaction with instructors and peers, learning outcomes that match expectations, services, and orientation.
Process/practice	Faculty/learner interaction is timely and substantive. Adequate and fair systems assess course learning objectives; results are used for improving learning.
Metric	See above and/or interviews. Alumni surveys, referrals, testimonials; focus groups; faculty/mentor/advisor perceptions.
Progress indices	Satisfaction measures show continuously increasing improvement. Institutional surveys, interviews, or other metrics show that satisfaction levels are at least equivalent to those of other delivery modes for the institution.

Adapted from The Sloan Consortium (2012).

Framework for Assessing Outcomes and Practices in Web-Based Courses in Nursing

This framework for assessing outcomes and teaching–learning practices in DE nursing courses (Billings, 2000) was developed from a review of the nursing literature about courses offered at a distance and integrates the Seven Principles for Good Practice in Undergraduate Education (Chickering & Gamson, 1987). The framework has three primary components and two supporting components. The framework begins with the outcomes that can be enabled by DE, such as learning (course- or program-specific); access; convenience; satisfaction; recruitment, retention, and graduation rates; productive use of time; preparation for real-world work; professional role socialization; and proficiency in using computer tools (computer literacy) and knowledge tools.

The outcomes are facilitated by teaching–learning practices that include active learning, time on task, respect for diverse talents and ways of learning, high expectations, prompt feedback, student–faculty interaction, and collaboration among peers. Effective teaching and learning in DE courses and programs are dependent on faculty and student development for teaching and learning as well as orientation to the use of the technology and ongoing technical and course/program support, motivated and rewarded faculty, and access to learning resources and services. The framework, therefore, also includes these variables as influencing teaching–learning practices. The third component of the model is the use of the technology, including technology infrastructure and user support.

Community of Inquiry

This framework is derived from the premise that an educational experience is dependent on interaction among the participants (Effken, 2008; Garrison, Anderson, & Archer, 2000; Mayne & Wu, 2011; Rourke, Anderson, Garrison, & Archer, 2001). The model consists of three "presences"—social presence, cognitive presence, and teaching presence—which converge during an educational experience and promote learning. Social presence, the ability of the participants (students and faculty) to present themselves as real people and to feel connected to the members in the online community, leads to an increased perception of participating in a community, fosters interaction, and ultimately leads to other outcomes such as retention and satisfaction (Effken, 2008; Mayne & Wu, 2011). Cognitive presence refers to the inquiry and critical thinking that is promoted through interaction in the community, and teaching presence is established through the design and development of the course along with the faculty's ability to facilitate dynamic interaction.

Quality Matters™

Quality Matters (www.qmprogram.org) is an external, peer-review service that reviews courses using established standards and rubrics and makes suggestions for improvement in the design of the course. The standards and rubric for 2011–2013 are located at www.qmprogram.org/files/QM_Standards_2011-2013.pdf. The standards used for review of courses include Overview and Introduction, Learning Objectives (Competencies), Assessment and Measurement, Instructional Materials, Learner Interaction and Engagement, Course Technology, Learner Support, and Accessibility. The review of literature behind the standards is extensive (www.qmprogram.org/files/rubric/appendix.pdf), and schools of nursing or their parent institutions can subscribe to the service.

QM PROCESS

QM is an ongoing process (Chao, Saj, & Tessier, 2006). Similar to other evaluation and research processes, QM involves determining the purpose for the QM, identifying the objective(s) of the inquiry, specifying a time frame, selecting who should be involved in the monitoring process, selecting a framework to guide the evaluation (if appropriate) and related instruments and methods, and using the findings to improve the DE program or course. The ultimate purpose of all QM efforts is to improve the DE course or program. Identifying the purpose of the QM broadly is useful when DE is being first implemented, but as the students, faculty, administrators, and technical support team become more experienced in offering courses and programs, the purpose may be narrowed to target specific aspects of the program for monitoring and improvement.

Writing down the objectives for QM adds focus and clarity and guides subsequent decisions about what indicators of quality to monitor. Since there are many aspects of a DE program to monitor, it is helpful to limit the scope to focus on questions that are of immediate concern or where changes can be made quickly if needed. During initial offerings of a program or course, it may be more important to focus on student orientation, faculty preparation, use of technology, and design and navigation of the courses. As the DE offerings mature, the focus may shift to gathering information about learning outcomes, student retention, and preparation for practice roles.

At the outset, educators should specify the time frame for gathering data about the course or program. Formative evaluation provides information for immediate change, while gathering data at the end of courses, semesters, or programs (summative evaluation) provides information about long-term outcomes. As with all evaluation efforts, gathering too much information, information that cannot be used to effect change, or information about processes that cannot be changed wastes resources. Chao, Saj, and Tessier (2006) recommend a sampling procedure when evaluating large programs with many courses whereby not every course is reviewed every year.

As with course and program evaluation for on-campus courses, many stakeholders must be included in QM for DE. In addition to students, faculty, administrators, accrediting agencies, funders, and campus program review committees, the QM team for DE courses and programs should also include instructional designers, registrars, website designers, providers of course-management systems, and technology support staff members who were involved in the course delivery. Evaluators may be internal to the school of nursing or contracted to provide external review. External evaluators, such as the Quality Matters program, provide unbiased feedback. Institutional review panels (internal) and accrediting agencies (external) also are key evaluators in the QM process.

As with all course development and teaching, faculty must obtain feedback from students about teaching and course effectiveness and use it to continuously improve course quality (Chao, Saj, & Tessier, 2006). Colleagues are also helpful in providing feedback about course or program quality. Peer review of web courses is another way to receive feedback about the course design and impact on student learning (Cobb et al., 2001). Peer review may include informal review of the course and teaching by colleagues and integrating suggestions for improvement. Zsohar and Smith (2008) suggest that peer reviewers have experience and expertise teaching online as well as the necessary content expertise, and that they use pre-established criteria for evaluating the course and instruction. Another review method is to invite colleagues outside nursing but with online teaching experience to review the course. Review that is more formal occurs when peers review courses for promotion, tenure, or teaching awards.

Framework, Methods, and Instruments to Guide QM

Frameworks offer the advantage of organizing the quality indictors into a model that can link several quality indicators and show relationships among them. Using a testable framework for assessing DE programs has many advantages for nurse educators. A framework guides assessment of outcomes and interventions taken to improve DE programs and informs judgments about allocation of resources. A framework also lends rigor to assessment efforts by guiding analysis of the findings of the assessment of DE in nursing, identifying gaps in the research, and selecting appropriate variables for future study. Finally, using a common framework can assist nurse educators in understanding the impact of the use of technology on teaching and learning. The Framework for Assessing Outcomes and Practices in Web-Based Courses in Nursing (Billings, 2000; Billings, Connors, & Skiba, 2001) and the Community of Inquiry model (Mayne & Wu, 2011) are two examples of such frameworks.

A variety of methods can be used in QM, including descriptive studies, qualitative methods, and benchmarking. Descriptive studies using questionnaires have been a common approach to conducting QM. Qualitative approaches such as interviews and focus groups are helpful in eliciting information and were used in many early studies on DE (Mancuso-Murphy, 2007). Benchmarking is another method used to improve practices by mapping practices used in one setting against practices considered the gold standard in another, but similar, setting (Billings, Skiba, & Connors, 2005).

Educators create or use available instruments to gather data for QM activities. Faculty-developed questionnaires/surveys are used in QM activities. Users must establish reliability and validity of the instrument. Instruments that have been reported in the literature include the social presence scales (Brownrigg, 2005; Mayne & Wu, 2011), group interaction scales (Mayne & Wu, 2011), and the Evaluating Educational Uses of the Web in Nursing (EEUWIN) benchmarking instrument (Billings, Connors, & Skiba, 2001; Billings, Skiba, & Connors, 2005).

Course evaluations solicited from students/participants may be standardized to meet school of nursing, campus, or agency requirements. Course evaluation instruments used for monitoring quality in on-campus courses need to be modified for DE or at least have a section of questions added that elicit the specific information required to answer QM questions. Findings from course evaluations are used to improve course quality (Chao, Saj, & Tessier, 2006), and it is helpful when faculty inform students of the changes made based on the students' evaluation of the course. Gathering data from participants in DE courses can be simplified by using electronic survey instruments or those offered in the course-management system set up as an anonymous survey. There are also no-cost and low-cost online survey services such as SurveyMonkey® (www.surveymonkey.com) and FreeOnlineSurveys (freeonlinesurveys.com).

The primary purpose of any form of QM should be to judge the merit or the worth of whatever is being monitored. This applies to student learning outcomes from a course or program, the instructional activities of the faculty member, the design of a particular course, and the medium used either as an adjunct or as a delivery method for a specific course or program. Data collected through the evaluation process for DE courses must be used for making rational decisions and ultimately involves faculty, administrators, and the various stakeholders.

Data collected and analyzed within courses and program can be used to make a variety of evidence-based decisions. Decisions on effective and efficient use of student and faculty time, faculty workload issues, promotion and tenure issues, merit-raise concerns, and ethical and proprietary issues (i.e., who "owns" the course[s]) require data. Additional decisions requiring data include measuring costs related to course-delivery methods; student costs related to traveling to additional sites (for orientation, "immersion," testing, or blended/hybrid courses that require on-campus time); and costs for equipment (computers, broadband access, web cameras).

ACCREDITATION IN NURSING DE

Accreditation by appropriate bodies communicates to students, employers, community members, funding sources, and other interested and invested persons that quality measures are in place and are evaluated, and that preferred outcomes are met. While accreditation for nursing programs is voluntary, significant consequences arise when accreditation is not achieved. Colleges and universities do expect that educational units are accredited by the appropriate body, and failure to achieve accreditation can have serious financial and administrative consequences. Additionally, lack of accreditation results in the inability of students to obtain many forms of financial aid, may inhibit acceptance into graduate programs, and may prohibit licensure and certification. Nursing programs that have earned accreditation have validation that quality standards are being met, both in terms of the processes of education and in education outcomes.

The U.S. Department of Education (USDOE) identifies two types of accreditation: One is for the institution as a whole, referred to as *institutional*, and the second is more focused, being *specialized* or *programmatic*. Nursing programs can achieve specialized accreditation through the National League for Nursing Accrediting Commission (NLNAC) or the Commission on Collegiate Nursing Education (CCNE). Some programs are dually accredited. The USDOE has officially recognized both the NLNAC and the CCNE as specialty accrediting bodies for nursing programs (USDOE, n.d.). Each accreditation body has standards and criteria required for accreditation. Nursing programs demonstrate meeting standards by developing a self-study document and by having an on-site evaluation from peers visiting the campus from the accrediting body.

NLNAC

The NLNAC has the authority to assess and award or deny specialized nursing program accreditation for postsecondary and higher education in practical nursing, diploma, BSN, MSN, and clinical doctorate programs both online and on campus. It is recognized as an accrediting body for all types of nursing education programs by the USDOE and the Council for Higher Education Accreditation (CHEA) among others (NLNAC, 2012).

The NLNAC describes the procedure and approval criteria for NLNAC-accredited nursing programs that wish to incorporate distance learning into the present program(s). A substantive change request and a minimum of 4 months' notice are required before implementing the changes. Approval is dependent on meeting critical elements: "congruence with the governing organization's mission; instructional design and delivery method of the course(s); preparation and competency of the faculty; quality and accessibility of the support services; accessibility, currency, and relevancy of learning resources; currency and appropriateness of the offerings relative to the method of delivery; provision for the faculty–student and student–student interactions; and ongoing evaluation of student learning, and provision for verification of student identity" (NLNAC Accreditation Manual, 2012, p. 51).

Standards and criteria for initial accreditation and re-accreditation apply to every nursing program and require programs to self-evaluate their performance on the standards. Each standard has an additional criterion related to DE. The last publication of standards was in 2008 and is located at www.nlnac.org/manuals/Manual2008.htm. Additionally, Standard 3 Criterion 7 is highly relevant to distance learning and applies to programs online or on campus: "Orientation to technology is provided and technological support is available to students including those receiving alternative methods of delivery" (NLNAC Accreditation Manual, 2012, pp. 71, 77, and 83).

Before and during a site visit by the accrediting agency, access to all of the DE materials is made available to the site evaluation team. The classes (current and past), student orientation, faculty orientation, library, student services, and other materials are reviewed at the time of the site visit. For courses, evaluators examine the syllabi, course, and unit objectives, class grades, discussion questions, faculty interactions with students, assignment feedback, and grading rubrics. For the program, evaluators will examine technology and program orientation materials for students and faculty, policies related to the DE courses such as identification of student identity, late policies, attendance policies, and technology support services. Policies and services for DE students must be equivalent to the services for on-campus students.

CCNE

The CCNE was established in 1996, arising from the work of the American Association of Colleges of Nursing (AACN) to establish an accrediting body for nursing programs in universities and 4-year colleges. CCNE accredits programs offering bachelor's, master's, and doctoral degrees as well as nurse residency programs (CCNE, 2009). In the series of documents *The Essentials*, CCNE provides guidance for curriculum and expected educational outcomes specific to each program type (AACN, 2012). Arising from *The Essentials* are standards and key elements for each program type, including mission and governance, institutional commitment and resources, curriculum and teaching–learning practices, and program effectiveness.

The same level of quality and program outcomes is expected from distance-learning programs as from on-campus classrooms. CCNE supports the Alliance for Nursing Accreditation (2002) statement on distance learning, which is endorsed by other major nursing organizations, including the National Council of State Boards of Nursing (NCSBN). "All nursing education programs delivered solely or in part through distance-learning technologies must meet the same academic program and learning support standards and accreditation criteria as programs provided in face-to-face formats" (CCNE, 2007). CHEA published findings in 2002 about the standards used for measuring the quality of DE programs (CHEA, 2002).

Though the CCNE standards and key elements do not differ for distance-learning programs, the process by which these standards are met and the evidence required to meet the standards may require additional effort. For example, Standard I, Program Quality: Mission and Governance Key Element I-D, states that faculty and students should participate in program governance. Programs would need to create both the technical support and the atmosphere of engagement necessary to include distance-learning students in committee memberships and other opportunities for participation in decision making. The key elements in Standard II, Program Quality: Institution Commitment, speak to fiscal and physical resources, support for teaching and learning in the online environment, and the preparation of the faculty. Support from information technology services, involvement of instructional design experts, and the ongoing education of faculty in delivery of DE should be carefully planned, implemented, and evaluated in view of the needs of the DE program and the needs of the students. In responding to Standard III, Program Quality: Curriculum and Teaching–Learning Practices, nursing programs show how the instructional process in their DE courses and programs meets the educational needs of their students. Examples of asynchronous and synchronous learning activities can demonstrate how students with various learning styles can be supported in online courses. Standard IV, Program Effectiveness: Student Performance and Faculty Accomplishments, are addressed in the same manner for DE programs as for on-campus programs. However, as noted early in the chapter, instruments that can measure the satisfaction with DE classes, social presence scales, or group interaction scales, may be needed.

The USDOE has certified several organizations that offer accreditation at the institutional level. Colleges and universities that provide postsecondary education, for Title IV participation, may seek accreditation through one of the six regional accrediting organizations recognized by the USDOE (n.d.), which are the Middle States Association of Colleges and Schools, New England Association of Schools and Colleges, North Central Association of Colleges and Schools, Northwest Accreditation Commission, Southern Association of Colleges and Schools, and Western Association of Schools and Colleges. Another option for institutional accreditation is the Distance Education and Training Council Accrediting Commission (DETC, 2012), which currently accredits 110 public, private, and international DE institutions.

State Boards of Nursing

When considering offering DE programs in nursing, keeping up with 50 state boards of nursing is also a challenge. In some states, the boards of nursing may create additional regulations for distance nursing programs. The Arizona Board of Nursing provides regulations for out-of-state DE nursing programs (Arizona Board of Nursing, 2012). Extra caution is to be used even with blended instruction, as the California Board of Nursing posted this on its website: "The Board has not approved any distance-learning programs. Even if a nursing school is appropriately accredited by its own state or country, completion of a distance-learning program and/or blended instruction will not qualify an applicant to sit for the NCLEX®" (California Board of Vocational Nursing, 2012). This applies to both LVN and RN DE programs. Additionally, the NCSBN is very interested in DE nursing programs (www.ncsbn.org).

State and Federal Oversight of DE

Oversight and regulation of DE on the state level is inconsistent. Some states have strict approval processes and oversight, while others leave concerns about appropriateness and quality to the individual institutions. Some states have marked differences between the requirements for public and private educational institutions. Concern about the lack of consistency has resulted in attention from the federal level. Requirements proposed at the federal level are tied to federal funding for education, including student financial aid. For example, Indiana State University has this statement at the bottom of their web page: "Distance Education Students Residing Outside of Indiana: Each of the states has its own approval processes for out-of-state institutions offering distance education. While Indiana State University endeavors to offer all of its programs to as wide an audience as possible, all ISU distance education programs may not be available in all states" (Indiana State University, 2012).

In October 2010, the USDOE issued regulations, one of which has a significant impact on DE: The State Authorization Regulation, Chapter 34, § 600.9(c) (WCET Advance, 2012). One aspect of this regulation would require that postsecondary institutions having distance-learning students meet the state requirements regulating distance learning in the state where the student resides. The institution in which the student is enrolled would be required to provide documentation of compliance with state regulations upon request of the secretary of state in the student's state of residence (Foxx, 2012). It would be possible for an institution offering distance-learning courses across state lines to be required to follow this process in multiple states, up to 50. This regulation was vacated in July 2011 by the U.S. District Court of the District of Columbia. While the USDOE is appealing this decision, Congresswoman Virginia Foxx (R-NC) introduced a bill, HR 2117, to repeal this and one other regulation begun by the USDOE. This bill passed the U.S. House of Representatives on February 28, 2012 (Foxx, 2012). U.S. Senators Burr and Nelson introduced S. 1297, the Senate counterpart of the House bill (GovTract.us, March 1, 2012). It should be noted that many organizations concerned with the quality of education supported the passage of HR 2117, including CCNE (Broad, 2011).

At the time of this writing, the complex issue of federal regulation of DE is volatile, with valid arguments on both sides. Applications of such regulations are of concern due to the complexity of its application and the burden on both the states and the educational institutions. Those who oppose federalization desire to preserve the latitude to make the decisions appropriate to individual states. Those who hope to see stronger central regulation fear a lack of consistency in quality, problems with consumer protection, and improperly managed growth and competition. More information about the state-by-state requirements can be found at wcet.wiche.edu/advance/resources (WCET, 2011). As the educational experience changes, so will accreditation and regulatory concerns and guidelines.

EXEMPLAR OF QM IN A DE PhD PROGRAM

The school of nursing at the University at Buffalo (UBSON) first offered a PhD in nursing degree program in 2005 and has completed the 5-year comprehensive program review at the university level. The program utilized the AACN quality indicators for research doctorates as the standard to monitor quality. The review showed the need for UBSON to create an innovative DE program to improve recruitment and maximize capacity of the PhD program. The Health Resources and Services Administration (HRSA) advanced nursing education grant funded for 2010–2013 helped UBSON develop the supporting infrastructure, engage consultants, and support faculty in preparing courses. The objectives of this project focused on improving the supply and diversity of PhD graduates by increasing access using DE technologies and pedagogies, increasing the overall enrollment of PhD students to 35, and increasing the retention and progression of PhD students.

Data supporting the decision to move to a distance-learning PhD program included requests from the applicant pool, assessment of current financial constraints, and the limited geographical access to high-quality doctoral education. Data from a past pilot DE program at UBSON helped to identify potential challenges, such as providing enhanced student and faculty supports and new strategies to increase access to PhD education. The use of the Community of Inquiry model was chosen to address the needs of doctoral learners.

The UBSON program is an innovative blend of traditional on-site and DE classroom learning that caters to local and international students who would ordinarily not have access to the program. Faculty and students meet yearly for summer orientations/intensives and at least once a year at national and regional conferences. The redesign process required instructional design experts to assist faculty in developing content and strategies to meet the course and program outcomes. The redesign of the courses was staggered over the 3 years.

The blended model includes both classroom instruction and videoconferencing within courses. In this way, students living in remote locations can access education through synchronous (videoconference) and asynchronous (online message boards and content) technologies. Local students participate synchronously in the classroom. The blended model is helpful to students who may be local but travel throughout the school year. The model also caters to those who enjoy online learning as well as those who prefer to be in the classroom.

The Community of Inquiry Model of Educational Engagement (CIMEE) serves as a framework for pedagogies that increase mentoring and socialization. This model is applicable for building a learning community that complements the DE environment and strengthens opportunities for mentoring students in the research scientist role. The CIMEE is a model that guides engagement in social, cognitive, and teaching presences. By design, social presence occurs in synchronous student-to-student and student-to-faculty communication to replicate the quality and informality of hallway conversations, in the form of a videoconference "virtual lounge" or in the classroom through formal presentations and interactions. Social presence occurs in face-to-face intensives, one-on-one videoconferencing, and videoconferencing for scholarly meetings or presentations. Cognitive presence occurs through the use of active learning strategies and technologies to explore topical issues and integrate previous knowledge with new knowledge. Teaching presence occurs through the design of courses that emphasize communication and facilitation of discussion and active learning strategies.

The overall evaluation of UBSON's program follows AACN's (2001) quality indicators for research doctorates. Focusing specifically on the DE component, the program used a combination of the Framework for Assessing Outcomes and Practices in Web-Based Courses in Nursing (Billings, 2000) to identify best practices, supports, and outcomes, and the CIMEE model to evaluate the learning process. Established surveys for each framework were combined to create an instrument used for primary data collection. This combined instrument was implemented through a web-based survey for each DE course. The results from the course surveys provide for ongoing program improvement within the comprehensive evaluation plan.

The evaluation plan includes a combination of primary and secondary data that measure the effectiveness of activities and objectives, including the implementation of DE methodologies, support resources, and evaluation of connectivity, and administrative record reviews to document the curriculum implementation process, recruitment activities, course evaluation strategies by students and faculty, and course grades. Other data pertained to student participation rates for programming and mentoring activities. Table 11.3 shows the specific project

TABLE 11.3 Summative/Formative Evaluation Outcomes, Measures, Responsibilities, and Frequency by Project Objectives for Quality Improvement (QI) and Overall University at Buffalo School of Nursing (UBSON) Measurement and Analysis

Project Objective	Outcomes/Evaluation Indicators	Measures	Frequency/ Responsibility
Objective 1: Increase access to PhD education for qualified nurses by using DE technologies and pedagogies appropriate to the needs of adult learners and courses with substantive content	1. DE technology systems identified and implemented	1. Student attendance report	Semester reviews/project director
	2. Support resources and processes implemented	2. Support resources in place	
	3. Student and faculty satisfied with DE orientation and training	3. Student and faculty training and orientation implemented	Semester reviews/project director
	4. Faculty implementing DE	4. Satisfaction surveys for faculty and students	Monthly analysis for QI/project director and faculty planning group
Objective 2: Increase to program capacity (N = 35 students) and maintain the current minority student diversity at 44%	1. Increase capacity to 35 students by Year 3; 30% increase from baseline	1. Admission/enrollment report	Each semester/ project director
	2. Student dissertation research funding sources identified	2. Student database of number of funded grants and publications	
	3. Maintain 44% diversity through targeted recruitment	3. Recruitment report	
Objective 3: Increase to 100% the retention and timely progression of all PhD students through use of the Community of Inquiry model	1. Less than 5% attrition for each cohort	1. Attrition report	Annually/ project director; project assistant
	2. Greater than 90% student satisfaction	2. Student satisfaction survey and spring and fall course syllabi and evaluations	Continuous quality improvement analysis at monthly project meetings
	3. Greater than 90% faculty satisfaction	3. Faculty satisfaction focus group and spring and fall course syllabi and evaluations	

(*Continued*)

TABLE 11.3 Summative/Formative Evaluation Outcomes, Measures, Responsibilities, and Frequency by Project Objectives for Quality Improvement (QI) and Overall University at Buffalo School of Nursing (UBSON) Measurement and Analysis (continued)

Overall UBSON Formative Evaluation Measurement and Analysis
Course evaluation: End-of-course student evaluations use tools developed by the UBSON faculty to measure student perceptions of course presentations, assignments, and learning achievements in addition to our survey tool. Faculty complete course reports each semester on overall effectiveness including recommendations for changes that incorporate student feedback. Recommendations for changes in curriculum as a whole are referred to the PhD committee and all faculty for review and approval.
CQI evaluation: The project director and staff conduct CQI analysis at monthly project meetings. The project assistant will implement CQI evaluation strategies such as (a) intensive and directive consultations with students at various times through their academic progression and (b) individual semester-based interviews with all students for feedback.
Tracking graduate performance: Students submit yearly annual reports that reflect their progress in the program, including research projects, grants, awards, publications, and socialization activities, which are summarized in a database in the UBSON Center for Nursing Research. The UBSON surveys all graduates regarding employment, publications, and grants and salary 6 months after graduation and every 5 years thereafter. The UB Graduate School also obtains satisfaction data from all PhD graduates in addition to the survey of earned doctorates upon exit.
Performance evaluation: Performance evaluation data are analyzed for all graduates, including grade point average (GPA), publications, grants, and employment after graduation, specifically employment as faculty in schools of nursing or research organizations.

DE = distance education; CQI = continuous quality improvement.

objectives and summarizes evaluation outcomes (evaluation indicators), measures, responsibilities, and frequency.

The PhD program has completed the first semester of courses for the first cohort that includes DE students. The midterm evaluation determined that students are overall satisfied with the courses. Distance students also valued the summer orientation intensive for building relationships among students. Program administrators agree that early application of the CIMEE supports pedagogical implementation and that Billings's (2001) model supports evaluation of best practices and outcomes. Both models have been helpful in identifying DE practices that are most useful and recognizing that transition to DE is an iterative process that requires structured supports for faculty and students.

SUMMARY AND KEY POINTS

QM in DE courses and programs is a comprehensive process that includes input from all individuals involved. As the use of DE in nursing increases, stakeholders will demand that evaluative data be collected, analyzed, reported, and used for decision making. This chapter has described the process and resources for monitoring quality in nursing DE courses and provided an exemplar of how one school of nursing has developed a system for monitoring its courses.

Key Points

1. DE in nursing education began in the 1980s and 1990s, and has evolved to include advanced QM techniques and frameworks.
2. Research findings show that DE is an effective method for providing nursing education. Finding from studies can provide evidence for making decisions about teaching-learning practices, methods and frequency of providing feedback from students and instructors, formation of professional identity and clinical reasoning, orientation to technology, learning resources, and the online community, and provision for student support services.
3. Faculty development in methodology for teaching at a distance and allotment of resources for the development of new materials and training are considered when developing DE courses.
4. Two national groups with accessible quality indicators are WICHE and Sloan-C.
5. Quality Matters is a peer organization that can evaluate and provide feedback for online courses and programs.
6. Three frameworks for assessing quality of DE include the Seven Principles for Good Practice in Undergraduate Education, the Framework for Assessing Outcomes and Practices in Web-Based Courses in Nursing, and the Community of Inquiry.
7. The QM process includes the following steps: Identify a purpose, write objectives for QM, specify a time frame, identify the stakeholders, establish process and outcome indicators, select a framework, identify the best data collection methods, create or use established instruments, standardize course evaluations, and analyze and apply the findings to improve future courses.
8. Accreditation by accrediting bodies in nursing education (NLNAC and CCNE) is voluntary, and established criteria must be met.
9. State boards of nursing are increasingly interested in DE nursing programs and quality.
10. State and federal regulations for DE have reached national concern. These require that nursing programs offered at a distance remain vigilant in the changing regulatory environment.

REFERENCES

Ali, N., Hodson-Carlton, K., & Ryan, M. (2004). Students' perception of online learning: Implications for teaching. *Nurse Educator, 29*(3), 111–115.

Alliance for Nursing Accreditation. (2002). Statement on distance education policies. Retrieved from http://www.midwife.org/siteFiles/career/Microsoft_Word_-_distance_ed_final.pdf

American Association of Colleges of Nursing (AACN). (2012). Leading Initiatives, The Essential Series. Washington D.C.: American Association of Colleges of Nursing. Retrieved from http://www.aacn.nche.edu/education-resources/essential-series

Anderson, K., & Avery, M. (2008). Faculty teaching time: A comparison of web-based and face-to-face graduate nursing courses. *International Journal of Nursing Education Scholarship, 5*(1), 1–12.

Arizona Board of Nursing. (2012). *R4-19-215. Distance learning nursing programs. Out-of-state nursing programs.* Retrieved from http://www.azsos.gov/public_services/Title_04/4-19.htm#ARTICLE%202.%20ARIZONA%20PROFESSIONAL%20AND%20PRACTICAL%20NURSING%20PROGRAMS

Bata-Jones, B., & Avery, M. (2004). Teaching pharmacology to graduate nursing students: Evaluation and comparison of web-based and face-to-face methods. *Journal of Nursing Education, 43*(4), 185–189.

Billings, D. (2000). A framework for assessing outcomes and practices in web-based courses in nursing. *Journal of Nursing Education, 39*(2), 60–67.

Billings, D. (2007) Distance education in nursing—25 years and still going strong. *Computers, Informatics & Nursing, 25*(3), 121–123.

Billings, D., Connors, H., & Skiba, D. (2001). Benchmarking best practices in web-based nursing courses. *Advances in Nursing Science, 23*(3), 41–52.

Billings, D. M., & Bachmeier, B. (1994). Teaching and learning at a distance: A review of the literature. In L. R. Allen (Ed.), *Review of research in nursing education* (pp. 1–32). New York, NY: National League for Nursing.

Billings, D. M., Skiba, D. J., & Connors, H. R. (2005). Best practices in web-based courses: Generational differences across undergraduate and graduate nursing students. *Journal of Professional Nursing, 21*(2), 126–133.

Bonnel, W. (2008). Improving feedback to students in online courses. *Nursing Education Perspectives, 29*(5), 290–294.

Broad, M. C. (2011). American Council on Education Letter of Support for HR 2117. Retrieved from http://www.acenet.edu/AM/Template.cfm?Section=LettersGovt&TEMPLATE=/CM/ContentDisplay.cfm&CONTENTID=41532

Broome, M., Halstead, J., Pesut, D., Rawl, S., & Boland, D. (2011). Evaluating the outcomes of a distance accessible PhD program. *Journal of Professional Nursing, 27*(2), 69–77.

Brownrigg, V. (2005). *Assessment of web-based learning in nursing: The role of social presence* (Unpublished dissertation). University of Colorado Health Sciences Center, Denver, CO.

Buckley, K. M. (2003). Evaluation of classroom-based, web-enhanced, and web-based distance learning nutrition courses for undergraduate nursing. *Journal of Nursing Education, 42*(8), 367–369.

California Board of Vocational Nursing. (2012). *Unaccredited nursing programs.* Retrieved from http://www.bvnpt.ca.gov/education/unaccredited_nursing_prgrams.shtml

Carruth, A. K., Broussard, P. C., Waldmeier, V. P., Gauthier, D. M., & Mixon, G. (2010). Graduate nursing online orientation course: Transitioning for success. *Journal of Nursing Education, 49*(12), 687–690.

CHEA. (2002). *Specialized accreditation and assuring quality in distance learning* [Monograph]. Retrieved from http://www.chea.org/pdf/mono_2_spec-accred_02.pdf

Chickering, A. W., & Ehrmann, S. (1996). *Implementing the seven principles: Technology as lever* [Online]. Retrieved from http://www.tltgroup.org/programs/seven.html

Chickering, A. W., & Gamson, Z. F. (1987). Seven principles for good practice in undergraduate education. *AAHE Bulletin, 39*(1), 306. Retrieved from http://www.aahea.org/bulletins/articles/sevenprinciples1987.htm

Chao, T., Saj, T., & Tessier, F. (2006). Establish a quality review for online courses. *Educause Quarterly, 29*(3), 32–39.

Cobb, K., Billings, D., Mays, R., & Canty-Mitchell, J. (2001). Peer review of web-based courses in nursing. *Nurse Educator, 26*(6), 274–279.

Commission on Collegiate Nursing Education (CCNE). (2007). Alliance for Nursing Accreditation Statement on Distance learning Policies. Washington D.C.: American Association of Colleges of Nursing. Retrieved from http://www.aacn.nche.edu/education-resources/distance-education-policies

Commission on Collegiate Nursing Education (CCNE). (2009). Achieving Excellence in Accreditation. Washington D.C.: American Association of Colleges of Nursing. Retrieved from http:www.aacn.nche.edu/Accreditation/index.htm

Coose, C. S. (2010). Distance nursing education in Alaska: A longitudinal study. *Nursing Education Perspectives, 31*(2), 93–96.

DeBourgh, G. A. (2003). Predictors of student satisfaction in distance-delivered graduate nursing courses: What matters most? *Journal of Professional Nursing, 19*(3), 149–163.

Distance Education and Training Council. (2012). DETC Accrediting Commission. Retrieved from http://www.detc.org/theaccrediting.html

Effken, J. (2008). Doctoral education from a distance. *Nursing Clinics of North America, 43,* 557–566.

Garrison, R. D, Anderson, T., & Archer, W. (2000). Critical inquiry in a text-based environment: Computer conferencing in higher education. *The Internet and Higher Education, 2*(2-3), 87–105.

GovTract.us. (March 1, 2012). S. 1297: A bill to preserve State and institutional authority relating to State authorization and the definition of credit hour. Washington D.C.: Civic Impulse, LLC. Retrieved from http://www.govtrack.us/congress/billtext.xpd?bill=s112-1297

Indiana State University. (2012). *Nursing (LPN/LVN to BS) bachelor degree completion program.* Retrieved from http://www.indstate.edu/degreelink/lpntobs/

Lashley, M. (2005). Teaching health assessment in the virtual classroom. *Journal of Nursing Education, 44*(8), 348–350.

Leasure, A. R., Davis, L., & Thievon, S. (2000). Comparison of student outcomes and preferences in a traditional vs. world wide web-based baccalaureate nursing research course. *Journal of Nursing Education, 39*(4), 149–154.

Lerners, D., Wilson, V., & Sitzman, K. (2007). Twenty-first century doctoral education: Online with a focus on nursing education, *Nursing Education Perspectives, 28*(6), 332–336.

Little, B. (2009). Quality assurance for online nursing courses. *Journal of Nursing Education, 48*(7), 381–387.

Mancuso-Murphy, J. (2007). Distance education in nursing: An integrated review of online nursing students' experiences with technology-delivered instruction. *Journal of Nursing Education, 46*(6), 252–260.

Mayne, L. A., & Wu, Q. (2011). Creating and measuring social presence in online graduate nursing courses. *Nursing Education Perspectives, 32*(2), 110–114.

Moore, J. C. (2011). The Sloan Consortium quality framework and the five pillars. Retrieved from http://sloanconsortium.org/publications/books/qualityframework.pdf

National League for Nursing Accrediting Commission. (2012). Home. Retrieved from http://www.nlnac.org/home.htm

National League for Nursing Accrediting Commission (NLNAC). (2012). NLNAC Accreditation Manual: Assuring Quality for the Future of Nursing Education.

Atlanta, GA: National League for Nursing Accrediting Commission, Inc. Retrieved from http://www.nlnac.org/manuals/NLNACManual2008.pdf

Nesler, M., Hanner, M. B., Melburg, V., & McGowan, S. (2001). Professional socialization of baccalaureate nursing students: Can students in distance nursing programs become socialized? *Journal of Nursing Education, 40*(7), 293–302.

Phillips, J. (2005). Strategies for active learning in online continuing education. *Journal of Continuing Education in Nursing, 36*(2), 77–83.

Pullen, D. (2006). An evaluative case study of online learning for healthcare professionals. *Journal of Continuing Education in Nursing, 37*(5), 225–232.

Rourke, L., Anderson, T., Garrison, D., & Archer, W. (2001). Assessing social presence in asynchronous text-based computer conferencing. *Journal of Distance Education, 14*(2), 50–71.

The Sloan Consortium. (2012). *The 5 pillars*. Retrieved from http://sloanconsortium.org/5pillars

United States Department of Education (USDOE). (n.d.). Accreditation in the United States. Washington D.C.: United States Department of Education. Retrieved from http://www2.ed.gov/admins/finaid/accred/accreditation_pg8.html

WCET. (2011). *State approval list of regulations for distance education: A starter list*. Retrieved from http://wcet.wiche.edu/wcet/docs/state-approval/FinalStateApprovalRegulationsforDistanceEducationAStarterListwithAddendum2.pdf

WCET Advance. (2012). 2010 federal regulations on state approval of out-of-state providers. Retrieved from http://wcet.wiche.edu/advance/state-approval

WICHE. (2011). *Principles of good practice*. Retrieved from http://wcet.wiche.edu/wcet/docs/tbd/TbD_PrinciplesofGoodPractice.pdf

Zsohar, H., & Smith, J. (2008). Transition from the classroom to the web: Successful strategies for teaching online. *Nursing Education Perspective, 29*(1), 23–28.

TWELVE

"There's an App for That!" Wireless and Mobile Computing in Distance Education

JEANNE P. SEWELL

WIRELESS COMMUNICATION TOOLS AND MOBILE COMPUTING

Mobile computing has taken us all by storm. It is everywhere: smartphones, tablets, software applications (apps), text messages, Facebook and Twitter, iTunes® U, e-books, and wireless technology are found at home, in the classroom, and in clinical settings. Selection and use of mobile computing in nursing education should be based on the desired outcomes for students. The cost and availability of the services should also be taken into consideration. Nursing students are facing a wireless world. Educators must stay abreast of current technologies used in the online classroom.

Smartphones and Tablets

Smartphones and tablets provide the ability to access e-mail, surf the Web, and use references and learning resources at the fingertips of the users. With numerous choices available, it is important to have an understanding of how the devices are alike and different. All smartphones can connect to the Internet using cellular subscription services and wireless (Wi-Fi) connections. All of the tablets can connect to the Internet using a Wi-Fi connection, and some of them also connect using cellular services. Cellular services in the United States usually require a user to sign a 2-year renewable contract for smartphones. Cellular services to support a tablet vary according to the usage but usually are only 30 days and renewable.

Smartphones

In addition to having the ability to make phone calls, smartphones provide access to Web sites and a variety of computer applications (apps) such as e-mail, word processing, an interactive calendar, and a calculator (Cassavoy, 2011). Different smartphones have similar features, but the specific apps are determined by the operating system (OS). For example the iPhone® uses the Apple® iOS, the Droids use the Google Android OS, and the Blackberry uses the Research in Motion (RIM) Blackberry OS. Smartphone users can download or purchase apps from the associated phone "store." Depending on the smartphone, users select and input information using a touch screen and/or a keyboard. The keyboard might be one with distinct keys or a virtual keyboard on the touch screen. Most smartphones also include a built-in digital camera, which can take still images and video.

Tablets

Tablets are popular mobile computing devices. Tablets refer to a device that looks like a slate. Tablets are usually larger than smartphones and come in a variety of sizes ranging from 4.4 × 2.23 inches to 10.4 × 7.2 inches. Tablets include all of the smartphone features with the exception of the ability to make cellular phone calls. Examples of tablets are noted in Table 12.1. The Kindle and Nook tablets began as black-and-white electronic book (e-book) readers, which also allowed the user to shop online for books. The iPad®, introduced in 2010, revolutionized the design of tablets when it offered a built-in camera, a high-resolution color display, full Internet access, and access to multiple types of apps,

TABLE 12.1 Examples of Tablet Devices

Produced for	Name of tablet	Sizes in inches
Amazon	Kindle	10.4 × 7.2; 7.5 × 4.8
Apple	iPad	9.5 × 7.31
Apple	iPod touch	4.4 × 2.32
Barnes & Noble	Nook	8.1 × 5; 6.5 × 5
Samsung	Galaxy Tab™	10.1 × 6.9; 7.6 × 4.8
T-Mobile®	Springboard™	7.48 × 5.08

including e-book readers. The newest versions of e-book readers offer many iPad features, for example, a color display, Wi-Fi Internet access, and an optional cellular service access.

Web 2.0

Web 2.0 is the interactive web that allows the user to create and modify web content. The term was coined by O'Reilly (2005) to describe an emerging interactive web contrasted to static web pages. Web 2.0 uses *cloud computing services*, which refers to working with an online computer application rather than one that resides on a personal computer. Web 2.0 supports social networking, such as Facebook, Twitter, blogs, social bookmarking, really simple syndication (RSS) feeds, and video and photo sharing. It allows users to create avatars and interact with others in virtual worlds. It also allows users to connect using VoIP (Voice over Internet Protocol) using telephone simulation apps such as Skype. One of the challenges with Web 2.0 is that it has emerged and morphed so quickly with few guidelines on best practices for use.

SOCIAL NETWORKING

Social networking allows us to connect with others around the world based upon interests. In addition to information and experiences, it supports the use of sharing media, such as pictures, videos, and audio. In other words, it is a "way to gather for conversation" (Petruniak, Krokosky, & Terry, 2011, p. 50). From a nursing perspective it provides a forum not only for personal use but also for therapeutic uses for patients and families. Examples are Facebook and Twitter.

Facebook

Facebook (www.facebook.com) is one of several popular social networking platforms. It was developed in 2004 by Mark Zuckerberg, along with cofounders Chris Hughes, Dustin Moskovitz, and Eduardo Saverin who, at that time, were all students at Harvard University (Facebook, 2011). Facebook was created to allow new ways for people to communicate. Other similar platforms include MySpace (www.myspace.com) and Bebo (www.bebo.com). These social networking platforms are available in many languages worldwide where there is an Internet connection. There is no fee for use, but users are required to create a log-in name and password. Social networking platforms are supported using advertisements.

Facebook is not only for individuals; the social networking platform has been adopted by organizations, such as nursing programs, universities, hospitals, businesses, and professional associations. A search tool allows users to find topics, for example, nursing, nursing education, autism, and diabetes. Users or organizations have "walls" where they can display a profile and where topics and photos are posted and others can make comments. Facebook also provides a way for users to post photos, send private e-mail, and chat.

Mesa Community College is an example of an innovative use of Facebook to support nursing education. Stella Bellman, a simulation manikin in the clinical lab, has a Facebook account (www.facebook.com/stella.bellman). Stella provides clinical tips and news and poses questions for nursing students. Her Facebook includes pictures of her family members (other manikins in the lab).

Twitter

Twitter (twitter.com) is another popular social networking tool. Twitter is similar to Facebook in that the service is free and users create a log-in name, password, and a user profile. Like Facebook, many businesses and organizations have a presence on Twitter. The difference is that Twitter uses short Tweets for communicating. Tweets, which can be no longer than 140 characters, provide a "pulse" on what is happening in the world with instant updates. Tweets, which can also include images, might have hashtags (# symbols) to note keywords. Tweets and replies are preceded with the associated Twitter usernames, which are preceded with the at (@) symbol, for example, @jeannesewell and @RWJF. Twitter Support includes an easy-to-follow guide with videos on how to Tweet (Twitter, 2011).

Twitter could be used in the online classroom with a learning activity where the students would search for a particular topic and then post it with a hashtag specified by the instructor. The students and instructor could search for the particular hashtag to compare the shared learning results. Twitter could be used to stay current with developing nursing topics, for example, the Future of Nursing (@FutureofNursing), the American Nurses Association (@ANANursingWorld), or the Institute for Healthcare Improvement (@IHIOpenSchool).

Blogs

Blogs, also known as weblogs, are searchable online commentaries that allow viewers to make comments. Some blogs serve as personal online diaries. Blogs may include graphics and videos, in addition to text. What distinguishes a blog from a website is the interactivity, as readers can post comments. There are numerous free blogging resources available (see Table 12.2). Blog platforms are free and include numerous choices of templates that can be personalized.

Technorati™ is a blog search engine. Users can search for blogs by category. The Technorati Authority uses a blog rating system to post the top 100 blogs every day (Technorati, 2011). Technorati provides a filtering service that limits searches to only blogs, unlike a standard search engine such as Google. Technorati allows users to search for topics relating to pertinent topics such as nursing or medical diagnoses.

Social Bookmarking

Social bookmarking allows users to save and store news articles and/or websites to a remote shared website and to share the sites with others (Gunelius, 2011). There are a variety of social bookmarking sites available on the web. All are free and require the user to create a username and password. Sites vary by purpose, so it may be appropriate to use more than one site (see Table 12.3). To learn more about social bookmarking, view this video: www.commoncraft.com/video/social-bookmarking.

Social bookmarking tools can be embedded in software designed for other functions, such as a citation manager. Zotero (www.zotero.org) is a free Firefox add-in or standalone that allows users to "collect, organize,

TABLE 12.2 Blogging Resources

Blog Name	URL	Features
Blogger	http://blogger.com	Free, customizable, numerous widgets, free themes, Google Analytics statistics, Google translator option
WordPress	http://wordpress.com	Free, customizable, free themes, numerous widgets
Posterous	http://posterous.com	Free, customizable, simple to use, designed for mobile blogging
Tumblr	http://tumblr.com	Free, customizable, free themes

TABLE 12.3 Examples of Social Bookmarking Sites

Site Name	URL	Features
Clipmarks	clipmarks.com	Allows the user create clips of text, images, and video from the web. The clips can be saved, e-mailed, blogged, or printed. Available as a web browser toolbar.
Del.icio.us	delicious.com	Online bookmarking for personal use and shared with others. Allows the user to organize sites by group. Available as a web browser toolbar.
Digg	digg.com	Features the best news, video, and photos as voted upon by Digg members. Users can contribute new sites, comment on postings, and save the sites for personal use.
Diigo	www.diigo.com	Online bookmarking that allows the user to save favorites, as well as highlight, clip, and annotate resources. Available as a web browser toolbar as well as an app for smartphones and the iPad.
Reddit	www.reddit.com	Allows the user to share and find new and popular news sites.
Slashdot	slashdot.org	Allows the user to post news and other topics for public comment.
StumbleUpon	www.stumbleupon.com	Allows the user to post and find websites based upon personal interests.

cite, and share" research sources (Center for History and New Media, 2011, para 1). The Zotero add-on citation library works only with the Firefox web browser, so it would work only on a mobile device that supports Firefox. Zotero includes a separate plug-in for word processors, such as Microsoft® Word® and OpenOffice.org, which allows the user to insert formatted citations with a click of the mouse while writing a scholarly paper and also to create an associated reference list at the end of the document.

The social networking feature in Zotero allows users to share the citations with groups on the Internet. The owner of the Zotero library can give permission to allow group members to add to and edit the library collection. Users can create an RSS feed (discussed later) to alert the member of any changes to the library collection. The library includes a discussion forum. Web browsers on mobile devices can be used to navigate to Zotero Groups, view the citations, and participate in group discussions. To visualize how to use Zotero Groups, go to www.youtube.com/watch?v=Bag6XdJIPLw.

Zotero could be used for group research assignments in the online classroom. Group members could search for journal articles and pertinent websites on a given topic. The results could be shared and discussed with other group members. Users could search for other groups researching the same topic to collaborate on research findings. The possibilities for using Zotero for collaborative research using mobile devices are endless.

RSS Feeds

RSS feeds allow the user to create personalized news feeds from the web, such as news, blogs, and podcasts, which can be received using an e-mail client such as Microsoft Word or a web page, such as iGoogle. Think of RSS feeds as the ability to design your own newspaper that arrives everyday. The ability to receive RSS feeds is built into most web browsers and news and blog pages (Pollette, 2004; USA.gov, 2011). An orange square button on the website or web browser means that RSS service is available. RSS may also be identified with an icon with the letters RSS or Atom, an alternative open-source form of RSS.

RSS feeds are written in XML (extensible markup language), which is similar to HTML (hypertext markup language). The XML provides the magic that allows the feeds to be shared. An RSS feed aggregator is used to display the information. A nursing instructor may choose to display an RSS feed in an online course by using an online, free RSS feed aggregator. All that is needed is the web address of the RSS feed and then the XML code output copied to a course web page in the HTML view. Feed2JS (feed2js.org) is an example of a free RSS feed aggregator. The website has easy-to-follow directions on how to use the aggregator to create an XML code that generates a RSS feed.

SHARED DOCUMENTS

There are a variety of opportunities to share documents in the online learning environment. Examples of shared documents include word processing, spreadsheets, slide shows, flashcards, and gaming activities. In some cases, the collaboration can be done simultaneously in a synchronous distance setting.

Two applications that can be used to share Office Suite documents on mobile devices are Google Docs and Microsoft Office Live SkyDrive. Google Docs is a free app and provides users with 5 gigabytes (GB) of free storage (Google, 2011). File size limitations vary according to the type of app. Users need only to have a Google account to edit documents; a Gmail address is not necessary. To learn how to create a Google account, view the video at www.youtube.com/watch?v=gJpkRbNto7E. Collaborative document editing can be done in real time in the synchronous environment. Documents can be shared with everyone or selected users. Google Docs allows users with a Mac or PC to create and share the following types of apps: document, presentation, spreadsheet, form, drawing, table (beta database app), and collection (see Figure 12.1). Currently, users with mobile devices are limited to creating and sharing only word processing documents and spreadsheets; however, they can still view other types of shared Google Docs files.

Microsoft Office Live SkyDrive (live.com) is free for users who have a personal copy of Microsoft Office 2007 or newer (Office 2013 will be available within the next year). Users have 25 GB of free file storage with a maximum file size of 7 megabytes (MB). SkyDrive is similar to Google Docs. Collaborative users with a Mac or PC can create; edit in real time; and share Microsoft Word, Excel®, PowerPoint®, and OneNote files (see Figure 12.2). Users with mobile devices can view and download documents from SkyDrive; however they cannot create files using Word, Excel, or PowerPoint. SkyDrive also allows users to upload and store pictures. For more information on how to share SkyDrive files, go to explore.live.com/

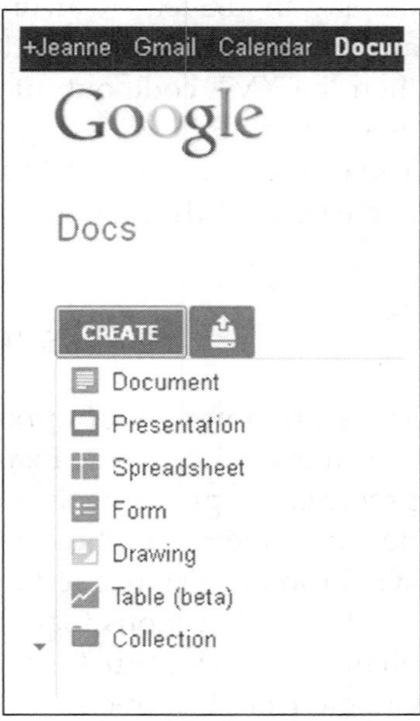

FIGURE 12.1 Google Docs.

FIGURE 12.2 Microsoft Office Live SkyDrive.

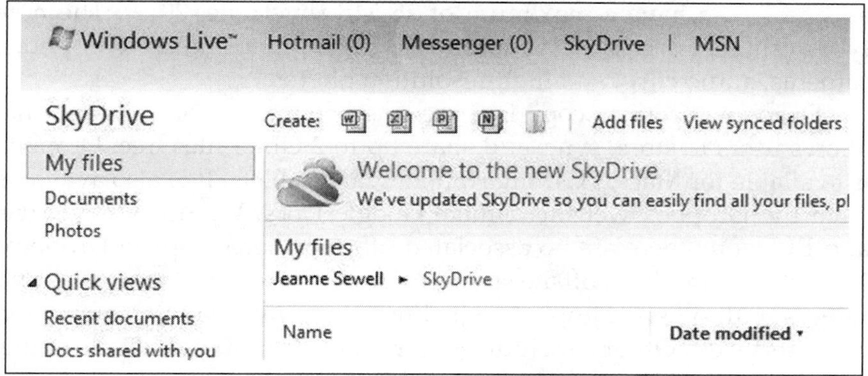

skydrive-share-photos-files?T1=t3. SkyDrive files can be accessed on smartphones and tablets that have a web browser and an Internet connection.

OneNote is a separate note-taking app that can be purchased for the desktop PC or downloaded from the mobile device store. OneNote allows users to create digital notebooks/binders and to share the contents with others. All of the Microsoft 2007 and 2010 apps can "print" to OneNote. When OneNote is opened, the files from other apps are available to be added to the appropriate digital binder. The notebooks can contain pictures, hyperlinks, scanned documents, and audio and video files (see Figure 12.3). For more information about OneNote, go to OneNote Help and How-To at office.microsoft.com/en-us/onenote-help. The OneNote app is available for the iPhone, iPad, and mobile devices that use the Microsoft OS.

Evernote (www.evernote.com) is a free cloud computing app that allows users to take e-ink and media notes and archive the web pages, pictures, and videos using mobile devices. Evernote is similar to OneNote. The notes can be shared with others using e-mail, Facebook, and Twitter. It is available for Macs, PCs, smartphones, and tablets and

FIGURE 12.3 Microsoft OneNote.

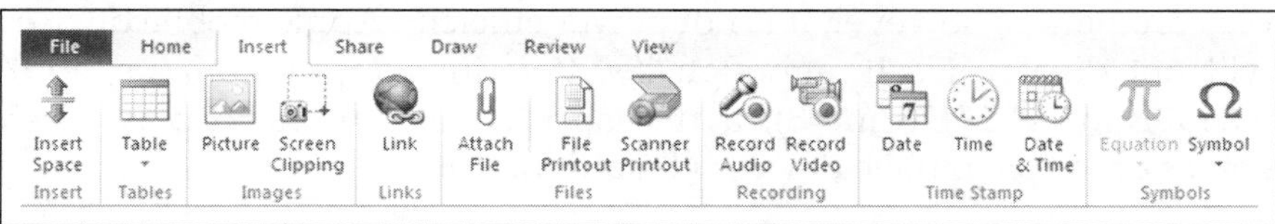

from the Evernote website. Evernote users can have 100,000 notes and each note can have a maximum of 25 MB (Evernote, 2012). The note types can vary across web e-ink notes, clips, photos taken with phone cameras, audio clips, and high-resolution photos.

Dropbox (dropbox.com) is a free cloud computing storage app that allows users to store, sync, and share up to 2 GB of files free. Dropbox is available for Macs, PCs, smartphones, and tablets. It is also available from the Dropbox website. Unlike Google Docs, Windows SkyDrive, and Evernote, there are no associated office or notes apps in Dropbox. It functions simply as offsite storage. Dropbox users can share files and folders with others. Dropbox is just one of many free file storage and sync services. Others include SugarSync, ZumoDrive, TeamDrive, and OpenDrive (Yang, 2011). Do a web search using "free cloud storage mobile" as the search term to find other solutions that will work with mobile devices.

Numerous other mobile device apps allow collaborative sharing and features useful to nursing students. For example, SlideShare (www.slideshare.net) allows users to upload, share, and search for slide presentations. The creator can choose to allow or disable the ability for others to download or embed the presentation on a blog or web page. Viewers can save the presentation as a favorite and make comments. Flashcards are another study tool that can benefit nursing students. There are many flashcard apps available for users of Macs, Windows PCs, smartphones, and tablets. It is easiest to do a Google search to find a flashcard app that meets the user's personal needs. It is important to note that the creators of the flashcards may be novice nursing students who have created cards with incorrect information. Just because the flashcards exist does not make the information valid.

Games are yet another resource that could benefit online learners. The creation or selection of the game is dependent upon the desired learning outcomes and the setting. Teaching Educational Games Resources (opencontent.org/wiki/index.php?title=Teaching_Educational_Games_Resources) is a wiki that instructors may find helpful. Hot Potatoes (hotpot.uvic.ca/index.php) and Quandary (www.halfbakedsoftware.com/quandary.php) are two free resources that allow users to create online educational games. Once again, the design and use of the games are dependent upon learning outcomes. Many games use Flash to display animation; however, it is not power efficient. Apple mobile devices will not display Flash, although iSwifter (itunes.apple.com/us/app/iswifter/id388857173?mt=8), a free app, enables users to play Flash games on Apple mobile devices (Takahashi, 2011).

VIDEO CASTING

Video casting refers to self-made videos, either by instructors or students, for the purposes of education and sharing. There are several ways to create video: use a standard digital camera and switch it to video mode; use a video camera; use screen capture software; or use slide presentation software, such as PowerPoint or Keynote, and convert it to video. It is important to make decisions about the audio component to the video because some audio file formats can inflate the size of the video. For more information on video file format comparisons, go to "About Video Help" at www.videohelp.com/oldguides/comparison.

The ease with which the video is created depends upon the OS. When converting a slide presentation to video, the Apple Mac and iPad2® (second generation iPad) offer a relatively simple solution using a combination of Keynote® and GarageBand® or iMovie®. The iPad2 can be used to capture video using the forward-facing and rear-facing cameras. While most iPad video apps are not free, the cost of the three apps noted above used to create video is less than $20. To learn more about using the Apple apps, go to "Apple in Education" at www.apple.com/education/mac or read the blog "With iMovie on the iPad2, Video Editing Is Fun Again" at www.xconomy.com/national/2011/04/08/with-imovie-on-the-ipad-2-video-editing-is-fun-again/?single_page=true.

Creating video using the Windows OS is possible but often more complicated than using the Mac OS apps. There are several online services that will convert a PowerPoint slide presentation to video. Although some advertise that the service is free, usually the product is crippled in some way—such as displaying a watermark or limiting the output. CNET, an online technology magazine, posts recommendations for video software at download.cnet.com/windows/video-software.

A free video solution is to use TechSmith Jing (www.techsmith.com/jing.html) on a PC. Jing will allow the user to capture 5 minutes of video and audio (TechSmith, 2011). TechSmith Camtasia Studio (www.techsmith.com) and Adobe Captivate (www.techsmith.com) are commercial software solutions. In order to learn more about how to create video, search YouTube™ (www.youtube.com) using the search phrase "how to create video for YouTube."

AVATAR EXPERIENCES AND VIRTUAL WORLDS

The computer provides fascinating opportunities for instructors and students to interact with others in virtual worlds. Virtual worlds are simulations that can be a fantasy environment or a replica of the real-world environment. Virtual reality (VR) uses the concept of illusions (Sewell & Thede, 2013). Although the virtual world appears to be a game, it is not one. Virtual worlds use avatars to communicate. Behind every avatar, there is a person. Avatars have the ability to free people from disease and physical disabilities. There are many virtual-world environments. The website Virtual Worlds Reviews (www.virtualworldsreview.com) provides an overview of many of the popular sites, including a synopsis of what is provided and any associated fees.

Second Life is an example of a three-dimensional (3D) VR environment. It is a free computer program that is downloaded to the Mac or Windows PC. Users select an avatar and clothing and create a pseudonym. The avatar can fly, teleport, and even drive vehicles. Avatars communicate using chat, instant messaging, voice, e-mail, and video. Second Life developers can purchase islands and construct buildings using real money. To visualize the use of Second Life in nursing education without downloading the program, go to YouTube (www.youtube.com) and search using the phrase "Second Life nursing."

Second Life has been used in health care for instructional purposes. For example, Weiner, McNew, Trangenstein, and Gordon (2010) are using Second Life to teach nursing faculty how to work with human simulators. The virtual island, NURSIM4U, has an outpatient center, a nursing home facility, and several homes with plans to construct a conference center. Second Life has also been used to train physicians on how to deliver bad news to patients (Andrade, Bagri, Zaw, Roos, & Ruiz, 2010), as well as in disaster preparedness for public health (Hoffman, 2009).

However, Second Life can be problematic. Second Life is not designed for mobile devices. There is a learning curve while users learn how to get their avatars to walk, fly, teleport, and communicate. It is possible to experience predator avatars who bully others with offensive language and nudity. For those reasons, many colleges and universities have chosen to build their own virtual worlds without using Second Life. Others have made their islands available to only selected group members.

CONFERENCING

Computer technology has created opportunities for virtual conferences. Participants are able to communicate using the traditional plain old telephone service (POTS), cellular phones, and mobile devices with and without cameras. There are several types of conferencing possibilities, for example, phone conferences, video conferencing, and shared-computer-screen conferencing.

Phone Conferencing

Anyone with a smartphone, tablet, Mac, or PC can create conference calls using VoIP technology. VoIP uses computer technology to place phone calls between two or more computers and between computers to landline/cellular phones without the traditional phone service. Skype (www.skype.com) is an example of a popular free VoIP app. Skype can be downloaded to Macs, PCs, smartphones, and tablet computers. After the users create a log-in name and password, they can add other Skype members to their contact list, identify who is online, and make VoIP phone calls. The calls can be made anywhere in the world to users who have Internet access, and Skype software is free. The number of participants depends upon the Internet bandwidth. For example, users who have dial-up modems frequently experience dropped calls. Skype also provides the ability to instant message and exchange files.

Video Conferencing

Online classes are sometimes most effective in a synchronous setting. Webinar software is a great solution if it is available. Examples of popular webinar software include Adobe Connect (www.adobe.com/education/hed) and Collaborate (Blackboard.com). Webinar software provides the traditional classroom lecture experience. The lectures can be recorded so that students can replay them when studying. The webinar window can display the photos of participants who choose to use the computer camera. The webinar host can allow participants to "take control" of the webinar. That allows the participants to give oral and slide presentations. Webinar software includes the ability to have virtual rooms—one for the entire class and others for group work. Webinar software emulates the class participation of a traditional classroom because students can raise their hands to ask questions. Emoticons display emotion. Most webinar software allows for users to use a telephone to access the classroom and to use instant messaging.

Skype can also be used for video conferencing. Currently, the free version of Skype allows video conferencing for two participants. With the Skype Premium subscription, 3 to 10 people can participate. Skype video conferencing is possible on any mobile device with a forward-facing camera.

Shared-Computer Conferencing

Shared-computer-screen conferencing is a third type of conferencing. Join.me (join.me) is a free application that provides the ability to share a computer desktop. The host of the conference downloads a small application. When the Join.me menu appears, it displays a contact join number. The host then shares the nine-digit number with the conference participants. Join.me includes a chat feature and allows participants to take control of the remote computer. Join.me is a way for students who work virtually in groups. It also allows the instructor to troubleshoot computer or software problems remotely. Closing the application permanently closes the remote control capability.

TABLET AND SMARTPHONE APPS FOR NURSING STUDENTS

There are hundreds of free and low-cost apps available for Mac, PC, and mobile devices that could benefit nursing students. The selection of a particular app depends on the learner and the situation. For example, medical references are useful in both clinical settings and the classroom. Journal references are useful for classroom learning and continuing education. A few popular apps are noted in Table 12.4. Many of the apps are designed for the iPhone and iPad, but there is a growing number available for Android and Blackberry mobile devices.

Smart app shoppers look for bargains. Some of the apps are free for short periods. To find bargains, use a RSS feeds for news sites that review apps. Examples are CNET (www.cnet.com), TC Geeks (www.tcgeeks.com), TalkAndroid (www.talkandroid.com), Pulse News (market.android.com), and Blackberry App World (us.blackberry.com/apps-software/appworld).

iTunes U

iTunes U is an Apple initiative to bring educational content to learners—wherever the learner is located. iTunes U includes learning resources for kindergarten through 12th grade (K–12), colleges and universities, and Beyond Campus. The Beyond Campus section includes learning

TABLE 12.4 Apps Useful in Clinical Settings and the Classroom

Medical references	• Epocrates (www.epocrates.com/products/?CID=PPC-Brand-IMEpocratesPPC-Brand-Content12&gclid=CMnKy_mA36wCFQen7Qod-HElZsA): Online drug book. Includes pill images, pricing, and drug–drug interactions. • RxDrugs (www.skyscape.com/app/rxdrugs.aspx): Online drug book. Includes pill images and drug–drug interactions. • Nursing Central: Includes Davis's Drug Guide, Taber's, Diseases and Disorders, Davis's Laboratory and Diagnostics Tests, and test preparation for paid subscribers. • CoIM (itunes.apple.com/us/app/compatibility-injectable-medicines/id427602564?mt=8): Interactive resource for learning about compatibility of injectable medications. • Shots by STFM (www.immunizationed.org/?gclid=CIW2_b2A36wCFc2A7Qodzw1D8Q): Group on Immunization of the Society of Teachers of Family Medicine—Includes immunization information for children, adolescents, and adults. • MD ezLabs (mdezlabs.com): Interpretation of lab values. • iRadiology (itunes.apple.com/us/app/iradiology/id346440355?mt=8): Searchable database for radiology images with explanation of findings for each image. • AHRQ ePSS (epss.ahrq.gov/PDA/index.jsp): Electronic clinical preventative services.
Translator references	• English–Spanish dictionary (www.spanishdict.com/ & www.spanishdict.com/iphone): Text and audio translations of commonly used medical terms. • Translate (itunes.apple.com/us/app/google-translate/id414706506?mt=8 & market.android.com/details?id=com.google.android.apps.translate&hl=en): Google translator for most world languages. Includes an audio translation for many of the languages. • Verbally (www.apple.com/iphone/from-the-app-store): Useful for people who cannot speak but are able to click on words and phrases or type on a keyboard to express themselves.
Journal references	• New England Journal of Medicine (NEJM) app (itunes.apple.com/us/app/nejm-this-week/id373156254?mt=8): NEJM full-text articles, clinical images with descriptions, audio podcasts, and video podcasts. • Medscape (www.medscape.com/public/mobileapp?src=google&ef_id=Al5OoLKGyR4AAAcE:20111130185601:s): Includes over 4,000 free online full-text clinical articles, monographs, and pathology references. • PubMed Tap (itunes.apple.com/us/app/pubmed-on-tap/id301316540?mt=8): Search for citation from the National Library of Medicine.
Concept mapping	• Popplet lite (itunes.apple.com/us/app/popplet-lite/id364738549?mt=8): Concept mapping application that allows for the use of figures, photos, and video.
Collaboration tools	Whiteboard (www.apple.com/iphone/from-the-app-store): Whiteboard application that allows users to connect and draw together Join.me (join.me): Used for computer screen sharing and online meetings. Works with desktop computers and mobile devices.

(continued)

TABLE 12.4 Apps Useful in Clinical Settings and the Classroom (continued)

Study resources	• Eponyms (itunes.apple.com/us/app/eponyms-for-students/id286025430?mt=8): Learn medical terminology acronyms and meanings. • Flashcards (www.flashcardapps.info): A review of the many different flashcard apps.
Productivity	• Sonic pics (itunes.apple.com/us/app/sonicpics/id345295488?mt=8): Application for creating a movie with an iPad2 or iPhone.

resources from worldwide museums and organizations such as the National Theatre, China Education TV, and the New York Public Library. The member institutions have all completed an application process to have a presence in iTunes U. Learning content for the member institutions can be public or password protected. Most of the learning content is free and accessible to the public.

Users can access the learning content in iTunes U in two ways. The first is from the iTunes Store in the iTunes program on a Mac or Windows PC. iTunes U is a menu tab on the iTunes Store window (see Figure 12.4). The second way is the iTunes app on the iPhone, iPod touch, or iPad. The iTunes U menu has several options for filtering and selecting resources. Selecting an item opens up a video or audio podcast.

Because there are hundreds of thousands of items in the iTunes Store, the main search engine serves as a quick way of finding pertinent topics. As an example, when searching for nursing learning resources, if the term *nursing* is entered into the search window, all items tagged with the term nursing show up. Selecting "geriatric nursing" opens a new window with resources organized into podcasts, iTunes U, and books. "iPad How To's" by Apple includes about two dozen short videos on

FIGURE 12.4 iTunes U in iTunes.

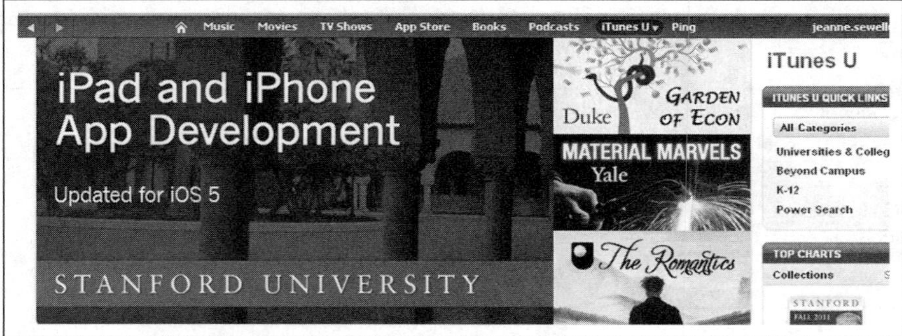

how to use iPad features and apps. The resources that "Viewers Also Downloaded" and customer ratios are located at the bottom of the window.

E-BOOKS NOW AND IN THE FUTURE

The ability to create and use e-books on mobile devices is one of the best opportunities for instructors and learners. e-books are commonly published as both digital books and audiobooks. As noted earlier, Barnes & Noble and Amazon first developed tablets so that their patrons could purchase and download e-books from their stores for use on the tablet. What may not be clear is that it is not necessary to have a specific bookstore-sponsored tablet to access and read e-books. Any tablet that allows the user Internet access and the ability to install new apps should be able to be used to purchase or borrow, download, and read/listen to eBooks from a variety of sources including commercial bookstores and public libraries.

There are several free e-book app readers available for all mobile devices (see Table 12.5). All of the app readers with the exception of e-books can be used with all or most mobile devices. As an example, Kobo™ offers a unique shared reading experience. Not only does Kobo allow users to purchase and read books, it allows users to share text passages to Facebook, have conversations with others reading the book, earn reading awards, and view reading statistics. Kindle also allows the reader to share reading with Facebook and Twitter.

TABLE 12.5 Examples of e-book Reader Apps

Produced By	Reader App	URL
Amazon	Kindle	www.amazon.com/gp/feature.html/ref=kcp_ipad_mkt_lnd?docId=1000493771
Amazon Kindle	CloudReaders	read.amazon.com
Apple	iBooks	www.apple.com/iphone/from-the-app-store
Barnes & Noble	Nook	www.barnesandnoble.com/u/free-nook-apps/379002321
Bluefire Productions	Bluefire Reader	www.bluefirereader.com/bluefire-reader.html
Borders (now Barnes & Noble)	Kobo	www.kobobooks.com
Lexcyle	Stanza	www.lexcycle.com

Many of the traditional nursing textbooks are now available as e-books. Major sources for nursing e-books are Skyscape (www.skyscape.com), Unbound Medicine (www.unboundmedicine.com), and Pepid (www.pepid.com). Users can try out the e-books for a free trial period or download demos of the products. Nursing e-books are also available from the textbook publishers and online vendors such as Barnes & Noble (www.barnesandnoble.com) and Amazon (www.amazon.com). Some e-books are available as a subscription, and others can be purchased. The advantage of digital e-books is that they are searchable, interactive, and available on a single mobile device.

In addition to purchasing e-books, some are now available at most higher-education and public libraries. The e-book adoption process has been slowed by publishers who fear that the commercial e-book sales will drop (Kastenbaum, 2011). The e-books that are available from libraries are protected by Digital Rights Management (DRM)—the same as music. That means that just because the book is digital it does not mean that it is available in unlimited quantities. Borrowers may still have to wait to obtain the e-book of their choice. There will still be a limited borrowing period. Although e-book borrowing is still a complex process, online learners have a growing opportunity to have quality learning resources using a web browser, a library card number, and an e-book reader. For more information on checking out e-books for reading with an e-book reader, view the video at www.youtube.com/watch?v=7kpyOU9WJo0 or search YouTube for additional information.

Self-publishing an e-book might be an option for both the instructor and nursing student. Creating an e-book is as simple as saving a word processing file designed as a book with a table of contents and index into an Adobe PDF (portable data file) document. PDF files can be read with most of the reader apps. Users with Pages word processing software on a Mac (which will not work on the iPad) can create and *export* files as ePub documents. For more information on e-book file formats and compatible devices, go to the OverDrive Device Resource Center at www.overdrive.com/Resources/DRC/Default.aspx. OverDrive distributes digital media including audiobooks and e-books to libraries, schools, publishers, and retailers (OverDrive, 2011).

iBooks® Author, released by Apple in January 2012, is a free app for the Mac that allows users to create digital books with dynamic page designs that are interactive. As examples of interactivity, the books can include a variety of media (video or audio files); quizzes with feedback (e.g., multiple choice, multiple choice with an image, adding labels to an image); Keynote presentations (the equivalent to Microsoft PowerPoint); and 3D interactive images (McKesson & Witwer, 2012). iBooks Author works with only the iBooks2 app for the iPad. iBooks Author interactive books for education are termed iTextbooks. iTextbooks can be offered free (no ISBN number required) or for a fee (requires an ISBN number) not more than $14.99 from the iBookstore.

Another option, especially if the e-book needs to be available for purchase, is to use a self-publishing company such as Lulu (www.lulu.com) or CreateSpace (www.createspace.com). Smashwords (www.smashwords.com) and Scribd (www.scribd.com) are other options for publishing and distributing e-books. Self-publishing is easy (Carnoy, 2010) and may be a viable option for the online instructor or student.

CHOOSING CREDIBLE WEBSITES AND WEB TOOLS FOR USE IN ONLINE LEARNING

Choosing credible websites is often like finding a needle in a haystack. Using a systematic process and practice is important to expedite and enhance the quality of the searches for all online learners. Health on the Net Foundation (www.hon.ch) provides an excellent guide for users to determine website credibility. When searching for medical and health information, the display of the HONcode symbol provides instant credibility for the website. Although Health on the Net is designed for medical and health web sites, the principles apply to all websites.

- Authority: The qualification(s) of the author(s) are clearly stated
- Complementary: The healthcare website makes it clear that the information on the website supports but does not replace the health care provider/patient relationship
- Privacy: The confidentiality of the website user is honored and maintained
- Attribution: Sources and references used are cited and include publication information, dates, and where applicable, web addresses. The date that the web site was last modified is noted.
- Justifiability: Any claims relating to benefits from resources noted on the website are justified and can be proven
- Transparency: The site provides a way for users to contact the author or agency. This is often located in the "About Us" or "Contact" link.
- Financial disclosure: Information about organizations and persons who contributed to funding the web site are clearly stated
- Advertising policy: Advertisements are easily distinguished from the website content (Health on the Net Foundation, 2011)

Other considerations for choosing websites include the website organization, design, and navigation menu. When evaluating organization, assess whether or not the purpose of the site and the intended audience are clear. When assessing design, there should be strong contrast between text color and background for improved readability. Graphics should provide added value to understanding the concepts that are noted. Graphics should be supportive of ethnic and cultural values. All capital letters, if used, are for titles or for emphasis because the use of all capital letters is considered "shouting" in the computer world.

WEBSITES FOR DISTANCE LEARNING STUDENTS

Efficient online learning requires learners to be proficient in using a computer, keyboarding skills, office applications, and digital resource search skills. It is not uncommon for nursing students to have a misconceived idea of their proficiency in the use of computers and computer apps. Fortunately, there are several excellent resources available; for example, GCF Learn Free, Hewlett Packard (HP) Learning, Microsoft tutorials, and YouTube.

GCF Learn Free (www.gcflearnfree.org/computer) is sponsored by Goodwill Community Foundation International and provides tutorials on a variety of computer topics. The tutorials are all free. Users can select a topic, such as computer basics, for lessons, interactives, extras, and videos. There are multiple topics ranging from Internet basics and Microsoft Office apps to Apple apps and OpenOffice.org.

HP Learning Center (h30440.www3.hp.com/learningcenter) is also free. Users are required to create a log-in name and password to access the classes. As with GCF Learn Free, there are a variety of computer topics, and the learning resources are interactive. The difference is that HP Learning Center offers a wide range of topics that include subjects like Windows 7, photo editing, and computer networking. Successful learners can print out a certificate after completing a class. HP Learning Center sends e-mail to subscribers to alert them of new offerings.

Microsoft offers free online training for all Microsoft Office products (2010, 2007, and 2003) at office.microsoft.com/en-us/training/default.aspx. Each training module includes articles and interactive courses. The courses are self-paced and have clearly stated learning goals, practice opportunities, and tests. After completing the course, the learner can print out a Quick Reference Card for the application. The Microsoft training website now includes a game, Ribbon Hero, so that learners can practice using Microsoft Office app ribbon menus proficiently.

Lynda.com (www.lynda.com) is a commercial product with training videos on topics ranging from computer applications to computer devices, for example, the iPad and Android phone. Several of the training resources are free to allow users to visualize the value of the resources. The training resources are available as monthly and annual subscriptions for individual users and corporations. A LyndaCampus subscription is available for educational institutions. It allows all Lynda.com training resources to be available to students, faculty, and staff using a log-in to the school's portal or IP network (Lynda.com, 2011).

YouTube (hwww.youtube.com) has many outstanding learning resources on a variety of topics ranging from clinical how-tos—such as blood pressure, physical assessment and blood gases, and disease management—to office applications and computers. Users can choose to subscribe to specific channels. To find a specific channel, the user first enters the terms in the search window and then selects "Filter & Explore" > "Channels" from the menu. Since the videos on YouTube are self-published, users need to use the information for choosing credible websites to determine the value of the video.

MERLOT (Multimedia Educational Resources for Learning and Online Teaching; www.merlot.org) is a database with links to several hundred thousand learning resources, many of which have been peer reviewed. MERLOT volunteers, who are primarily educators, complete a GRAPE (Getting Reviewers Accustomed to the Process of Evaluation) Camp prior to being assigned to a discipline specific editorial board. Although anyone can search MERLOT, users are encouraged to create a log-in name and password to become members. MERLOT members can contribute new learning resources and lessons for existing resources, create "Favorites" folders, and collaborate with others with similar interests. MERLOT has thousands of learning resources pertinent to nursing.

Digital library search skills are invaluable to the success of online learners. Colleges and universities worldwide have journal citations, full-text journal articles, and e-books available to their patrons. Each library will have a website with information and tutorials on how to search for scholarly publications. Some libraries provide a way to chat or e-mail librarians for assistance. Libraries subscribe to commercial databases such as EBSCOhost and Proquest with the journal resources. EBSCOhost (support.ebsco.com/training/tutorials.php) and Proquest (www.proquest.com/en-US/support/training/materials.shtml) provide tutorials on how to search for resources. Like any of the skills that a nurses uses, proficiency comes only with practice.

SUMMARY AND KEY POINTS

Wireless technology and mobile computers provide endless opportunities for instructors and students to collaborate in the online learning environment. They can experience untethered access to learning using smartphones and tablet computers to access courses and learning resources on the Internet. Learning opportunities are not restricted to the constraints of brick-and-mortar classrooms. Learning is available 24 hours a day at the convenience of the student and instructor.

In conclusion, today's online learner, equipped with efficient and effective use of computer technology and the Internet, has a goldmine of opportunities. Wireless and mobile computing in distance education allows the learner access to classes, e-books, and online references from mobile devices at a time and point of convenience. Technology expenses and availability should always be taken into consideration when designing online learning activities. When the learner can access the Internet with a desktop or mobile device, there is an app to do just about anything in today's distance education setting.

Key Points

1. Web 2.0 has opened ways to collaborate using social networking apps like Facebook, Twitter, and blogs.
2. Cloud computing provides access to interactive and collaborative resources like social bookmarking tools, RSS feeds, and shared documents. Files that are backed up and stored on the web can be shared with others.
3. Web 2.0 features provide the ability to create and share video and to collaborate with others using avatars in a virtual-world environment. Conferences using VoIP telephone simulation, video, and a shared computer screen provide enhanced connection between distance learners and their teachers.
4. Many of the apps for desktop computers and mobile devices are free or available for a nominal fee. Examples of free or low-cost apps include medical, translator, and journal references. Apps also include concept mapping, collaboration tools, study resources, and productivity tools.
5. The iTunes Store allows learners to access iTunes U for educational content for Macs, PCs, and mobile devices. In addition to iTunes U, the iTunes Store includes podcasts and e-books.

6. The added value of e-books is that they are searchable and can be bookmarked, stored, and accessed using mobile devices, such as smartphones and tablets.
7. e-books can be self-published with personal computers and/or with the assistance of online publishers that extend self-publishing services in areas of marketing and distribution.
8. Online learning requires learners to efficiently use the Internet to discover credible websites and web tools. The learner must critically analyze websites before use to ensure that content was developed by people or organizations with proper authority and that the content is valid, accurate, and current.
9. GCF Learn Free, HP Learning, Microsoft tutorials, and YouTube all offer excellent learner self-help resources at no charge.
10. Resources like Lynda.com allow users to access video learning on topics including hardware, such as how to use an Android phone or iPad; computer OSs; and specific computer applications, such as Microsoft Word and Excel.

REFERENCES

Andrade, A. D., Bagri, A., Zaw, K., Roos, B. A., & Ruiz, J. G. (2010). Avatar-mediated training in the delivery of bad news in a virtual world. *Journal of Palliative Medicine, 13*(12), 1415–1419.

Carnoy, D. (2010). *Self-publishing a book: 25 things you need to know*. Retrieved November 28, 2010, from http://reviews.cnet.com/self-publishing/

Cassavoy, L. (2011). *Smartphone—What is a Smartphone—Definition*. Retrieved November 26, 2011, from http://cellphones.about.com/od/glossary/g/smart_defined.htm

Center for History and New Media. (2011). *Zotero*. Retrieved November 27, 2011, from https://www.zotero.org/

Evernote. (2012). Overview of account data limits. Retrieved August 15, 2012 from https://support.evernote.com/link/portal/16051/16058/Article/532/Overview-of-Account-Data-Limits

Facebook. (2011). *Founder bios*. Retrieved November 27, 2011, from http://www.facebook.com/press/info.php?timeline#!/press/info.php?founderbios

Google. (2011). *Google Docs: How it works*. Retrieved November 25, 2011, from https://docs.google.com/support/bin/answer.py?hl=en&answer=39567&topic=1361454

Gunelius, S. (2011). *Social bookmarking*. Retrieved November 27, 2011, from http://weblogs.about.com/od/blogginglossary/g/SocialBookmark.htm

Health on the Net Foundation. (2011). *HONcode: Principles—Quality and trustworthy health information*. Retrieved November 30, 2011, from http://www.hon.ch/HONcode/Conduct.html

Hoffman, L. (2009). *First responders meet Second Life: Public health goes virtual*. Retrieved November 30, 2011, from http://vimeo.com/5673125

Kastenbaum, S. (2011, October 26). *eBook lending: Libraries go digital*. Retrieved November 27, 2011, from http://www.cnn.com/2011/10/26/living/digital-libraries/index.html

Lynda.com. (2011). *LyndaCampus*. Retrieved November 30, 2011, from http://www.lynda.com/online-software-training/lyndacampus.html

McKesson, N., & Witwer. (2012). Publishing with iBooks Author O'Reilly, Sebastapol, CA: O'Reilly. Retrieved from http://shop.oreilly.com/product/0636920025597.do

O'Reilly, T. (2005, September 30). *What Is Web 2.0: Design patterns and business models for the next generation of software*. Retrieved November 27, 2011, from http://oreilly.com/web2/archive/what-is-web-20.html

OverDrive. (2011). *About*. Retrieved November 30, 2011, from http://www.overdrive.com/About/

Petruniak, M., Krokosky, A., & Terry, S. F. (2011). Social media provides tools for discovery: How to find value in social networking. *Exceptional Parent, 41*(9), 50–52.

Pollette, C. (2004, July 13). *How RSS works*. Retrieved November 28, 2011, from http://www.howstuffworks.com/Internet/basics/rss.htm

Sewell, J.P. & Thede, L.Q. (2013). *Informatics and nursing: Opportunities and challenges* (4th ed.). Philadelphia, Wolters Kluwer.

Takahashi, D. (2011, November 9). *Adobe's mobile Flash crash could benefit game streaming startup iSwifter*. Retrieved November 28, 2011, from http://venture-beat.com/2011/11/09/adobes-mobile-flash-crash-could-benefit-game-streaming-startup-iswifter/

Technorati. (2011). *Technorati top 100*. Retrieved November 27, 2011, from http://technorati.com/blogs/top100/

TechSmith. (2011). *Frequently asked questions*. Retrieved November 28, 2011, from http://www.techsmith.com/tutorial-jing-faq.html

Twitter. (2011). *Twitter basics*. Retrieved November 27, 2011, from https://support.twitter.com/groups/31-twitter-basics

USA.gov. (2011, November 21). *What is RSS?* Retrieved November 28, 2011, from http://www.usa.gov/Topics/Reference_Shelf/Libraries/RSS_Library/What_Is_RSS.shtml

Weiner, E., McNew, R., Trangenstein, P., & Gordon, J. (2010). Using the virtual reality world of Second Life to teach nursing faculty simulation management. . . MEDINFO 2010: Proceedings of the 13th World Congress on Medical Informatics, Part 1. *Studies in Health Technology & Informatics, 160*, 615–619.

Yang, Y. (2011, April 14). *Top 10 free cloud storage service for you to back up and sync files*. Retrieved November 28, 2011, from http://freenuts.com/top-10-free-cloud-storage-services-for-you-to-back-up-and-sync-files/

Index